RENEWALS 458-4574
DATE DUE

DEC 2 0	DEC 17		
JUL 19			
DEC - 5	APR 07		
NOV 1 1			
	AUG 01		
DEC 13	SEP 20		
	DEC 05		
MAR 0 4	APR 1 3		
NOV 0 6	AUG 18		
FEB 1 9	NOV 14		
FEB 1 9			
APR 19			
May 11			

GAYLORD   PRINTED IN U.S.A.

M

J

CREATIVE
ART THERAPY

CREATIVE
ART THERAPY

By

Arthur Robbins, Ed.D., A.T.R.

Assistant Professor of Psychology
Pratt Institute, New York

and

Linda Beth Sibley, M.P.S., A.T.R.

Art Therapist
Mount Sinai Hospital, New York

BRUNNER/MAZEL, *Publishers* • NEW YORK

Library of Congress Cataloging in Publication Data

Robbins, Arthur, 1928–
    Creative art therapy.

    Bibliography: p. 255
    1. Art therapy.   2.   Art therapy—Cases, clinical
reports, statistics.   3.   Child psychiatry—Cases,
clinical reports, statistics.   I.   Sibley, Linda Beth,
1948–   joint author.   II.   Title.   [DNLM: 1.   Creativeness.   2.   Art therapy.   WM450 R632c]
RC489.A7R6   616.8′916′5   76-3647
ISBN 0-87630-122-7

Published by
BRUNNER/MAZEL, INC.
64 University Place, New York, N.Y. 10003

MANUFACTURED IN THE UNITED STATES OF AMERICA

Preface

After long struggles to be recognized as a more significant partner in the field of psychotherapy, art therapy has finally made an important impact. In my 23 years in art therapy I have witnessed many new techniques developed by art therapists used in mental health centers, rehabilitation centers, hospitals, schools, individual practice, and education, as well as for the expansion of healthy growth potential in people involved in other settings.

Art therapists who pioneered in the field—Margaret Naumberg, Edith Kramer, Hanna Kwiatkowska, Elinor Ullman, Myra Levick and others—often had great difficulty being accepted as serious workers in the field of psychotherapy. However, the contribution of Robbins and Sibley indicates the competence and professionalism now associated with the degree A.T.R.—Art Therapist Registered by the American Art Therapy Association.

In this outstanding book the reader will find detailed expressions of varied art therapy approaches. One has to be extremely impressed with the sensitivity and compassion with which the authors have put this book together, with their emphasis on the necessity for the art therapist to be trained to function appropriately as a facilitator for freer expression and to be competent as a clinical interviewer and therapist. Important issues such as ego development, respect for the autonomy of the person involved in art therapy, artistic growth, meaning of symbolism and communications are thoroughly discussed.

The three parts of the book complement each other in an integrated fashion. Robbins and Sibley's case study selections are well chosen and offer a broad panorama of the everyday, creative work in this field. In these days of instant authorship, it is a pleasure to find such a degree of scholarly application as is found in this book.

Especially to be noted is the chapter on technique, in which the authors state, "an art therapy technique is a concrete implementation of theory introduced by the art therapist, at the appropriate time, to facilitate creative and therapeutic change." They offer us the most comprehensive listing of techniques to be found in any publication known to me. Each technique is related to function, material, population, purposes and direction to achieve the objective sought. I heartily agree with the emphasis placed on the point that technique "can be no substitute for a sensitivity to the specific population, relevant issues, goals, atmosphere and setting."

The spirit of this book is exemplified in the authors' statement that, "Aliveness comes with creativity."

LYNNE FLEXNER BERGER, A.T.R.

New York, N.Y.
April, 1976

Contents

Introduction

In this book we are presenting thoughts about the development of an art therapist's theoretical and technical competence to effect therapeutic and creative change with a variety of populations.

Art therapy as a process cannot simply be delineated by listing skills, methods, or functions. An art therapist starts from where she is anchored in the creative process, using a wide variety of therapeutic systems and integrating them with all her knowledge and past experience as an artist.

Within this framework, the art therapist may find herself functioning as a therapist on a psychiatric team, as a remedial expert within a school setting, or even as a club leader with an adolescent gang. The range and scope of this emerging profession potentially reach into many institutional settings and there is the opportunity to make significant contributions to the science of communications.

Our conception of art therapy is not confined to the therapeutic side effects of art education or the service of an ancillary member of a psychotherapeutic team. Rather we propose to enrich and broaden the field by incorporating the humanistic tradition of the artist who is concerned with authenticity, individuality and self-actualization within the environment. All too often, educational and therapeutic endeavors are directed towards coping and meeting societal demands. Hopefully, the art therapy practitioner can make use of adaption and behavior modification techniques and offer with these tools an atmosphere that will promote an inner sense of excitement, discovery, change and creation.

The purpose of this book is to bring together in one text the theory, techniques, and practical material that will aid the individual attempting to evolve into this new conception of a full-fledged professional. Although no book or introduction can fully prepare a student for every eventuality that will arise in the stress and turmoil of daily work experience, with the availability of the following material, it is hoped emotional and cognitive growth will come together and be more easily comprehended. Learning art therapy is an emotional affair which demands that one function on a number of levels at the same time. One is also required to transfer the individual creative process from the realm of materials to the realm of human relations.

The historical perspective offered in the first chapter will open the door to the enormous amount of supplemental material available to the student. Art therapy draws heavily from many disciplines—science, humanities, philosophy, mythology—all of which the student may become familiar with in order to make the highest and best use of herself.

In the second chapter we offer insights related to the emotional struggle one undergoes in attempting to master the integration of self and profession. Becoming an Art Therapist will perhaps be referred to frequently during the learning process. We hope this section will present a lucid and easily grasped overall perspective to the student who may at times feel flooded by intrapsychic and interpersonal pressure.

Central to our conception of art therapy is a blending of creativity and therapeutic practice. It would be a loss if the theory were not grasped and the therapist relied only upon intuition and spontaneous responses. A profession needs clearly enunciated principles and tenets to enable its practitioners to test out hypotheses and to communicate viably with peer professionals.

The principles by which we attempt to heal need to be constantly discovered and rediscovered as experiences become concretized and shared. We aim not toward a negative intellectual network that wards off fresh discovery and insight, but rather the possibility of reformulating old experiences and discovering new conceptions.

The chapters on Creativity Development and Imagery emphasize the role of the creative process both within the art therapist and within the therapeutic dialogue. Here we state a core premise of this text: Creativity development is our special strength and the distinguishing talent of an art therapist. This process is broken down into ego development, nonverbal communication and an ability to make crucial shifts in ego states. The art therapist works with introjects, imagos and induced feelings. The capacity to capture the locked-in energies of these forces is a result of theoretical understanding, training and personal growth.

The chapter on special Clinical Considerations is meant as a focused approach to particular patient populations and is not a substitute for a thorough understanding of personality dynamics. In practice, it will be necessary to consider particular characterological styles as they relate to the specific use of materials within a creative dialogue.

In any training program, Institutional Issues absorb a large portion of a student's energy and time. The problems are formidable; we do not even attempt to provide a full review of institutional management and change. We attempt to sensitize the reader to recurrent issues, stimulate his imagination as to possible solutions, and to encourage further investigation and work in courses that deal more fully with this topic.

Our Case Studies offer a full illustration of how theory and technique interact and how personal and artistic growth proceed concurrently. When we have the opportunity to view clinical experiences within a variety of settings and through the eyes of seven different art therapists, similarities and differences become obvious.

It is usually assumed that the art therapy student comes to a training program with the skills of an artist, and yet the psychology of art materials is rarely discussed. Little can be found in our literature. Much room for elaboration and research remains here for students with a predominantly psychological background. We are but opening the door in our chapter on Art Materials. It is hoped that this initial outline will evolve into an entire coursework for study from which we can all learn.

The art therapy student will no doubt be tempted to turn first to the chapter containing a compilation of technical aids which resulted from many interviews, questionnaires, and readings. Since there is a void elsewhere, we understand this temptation. However, this section has been placed at the end, because we are deeply convinced of the necessity of mastering theory along with achieving real personal development as the right road to fruitful application of technique. We are confident that as a student gains maturity in personal growth and in field experience, she will constantly be developing and creating an original repertoire of techniques.

Our field is exciting and mercurial now. We are aware that what we write today may be outdated tomorrow as new conceptions and developments are introduced. However, we hope to share an eclectic philosophical and practical foundation useful for present work and future growth.

Art therapists have an immense reservoir of energy, skills and creativity to contribute to the healing professions. We need a theoretical conception and a flexible role model, supported by knowledge and discipline, as preparation to meet complex professional challenges.

Acknowledgments

Creative Art Therapy represents the thoughts and experiences of many people. The Pratt Institute Graduate Art Therapy students have contributed each in their own way to the development of this text. Heidi Sparkes selected and co-edited the six case studies illustrating art therapy as practiced by student interns. Julie Joslyn Brown also collaborated on Imagery: Part II. We are indebted to her for both the rich written material and extensive work in preparing the photographic illustrations. "Deanna" deserves our sincere appreciation for her permission to publish the psychoanalytic case report and her openness in sharing the art therapy experience from a patient's point of view. Gilbert L. Gordon's contribution to this chapter represents only a small portion of his continual editorial, philosophic and moral support.

Thanks are due Frances Plonsky, Frances Kaplan and Ruth Obernbreit for their efforts in reviewing initial drafts and to Susan Barrows for her editorial skills in the final drafts. We are particularly grateful to the students and professionals across the country who shared their art therapy techniques. Special mention must be made of Pergamon Press for their permission to reprint, in a modified form, the chapters on Creativity Development and Imagery: Part I from *Art Psychotherapy: An International Journal*. Perhaps most of all, our analytic and clinical experience has constantly influenced the formulations presented here. Our last and warmest thank you goes to our families, lovers and friends for their patience, encouragement and ever-cheerful support.

A. R. and L.B.S.

Goldens Bridge
March 1976

COLOR
ILLUSTRATIONS

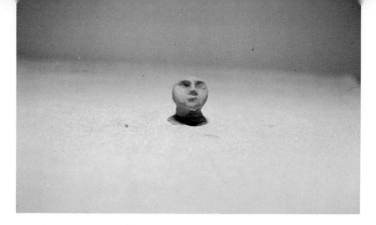

FIGURE 6.1: Initially the therapist misjudges Sam's level of functioning and relatedness and offers him a sophisticated clay image.

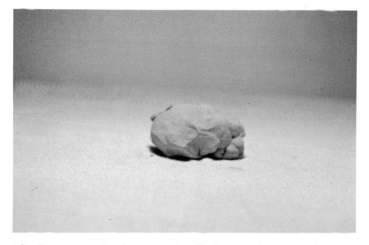

FIGURE 6.2: Sam responds with a primitively formed clay mass, clearly communicating his conceptual abilities.

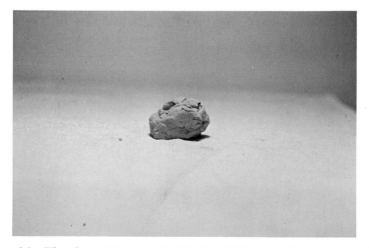

FIGURE 6.3: The therapist's second gift effectively states her understanding of Sam's form and content, serving as common ground for further dialogue.

B

FIGURE 6.4: The symbol of the woman/man functions as a catalyst. Sam acts out both destructive impulses and reconstructive efforts on the clay image.

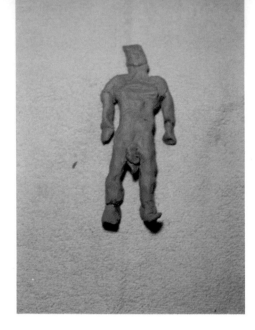

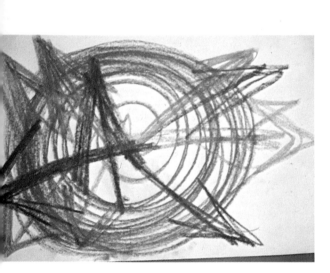

FIGURE 6.5: Davey's underlying terror and panic are felt by the therapist and appear in her drawing. The unconscious imagery accurately represents affects too threatening for either patient or therapist to acknowledge.

FIGURE 6.6: Again, the therapist's imagery captures the patient's unconscious attitude of hostility and sadism. Josephine recognized the therapist's painting as a reflection of her own feelings.

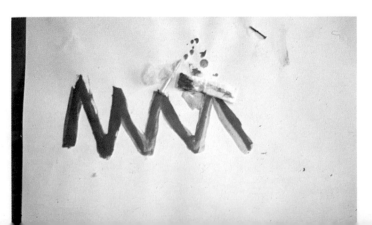

C

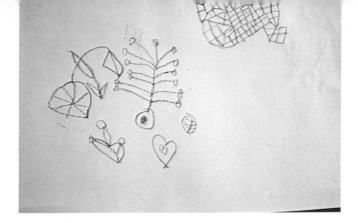

FIGURE 6.7: Josephine presents disconnected partial images that are tight, defended and yet hostile. Her verbal denial of such feelings was vehement.

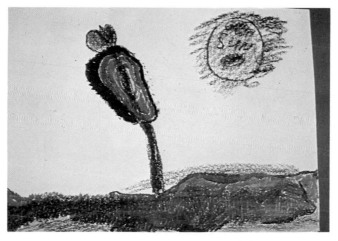

FIGURE 6.8: In a drawing by both patient and therapist, the art work functions as the vehicle whereby a symbiotic relatedness is played out. Josephine strengthens the connection between the "amoeba" and the "ocean," mumbling aloud, "osmosis."

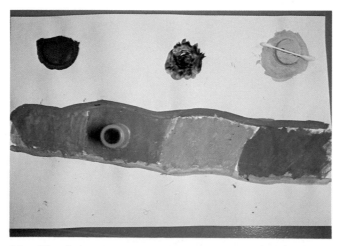

FIGURE 6.9: The therapist's "wall" (separation) was really Josephine's "railroad tracks" (individuation). While patient and therapist are equal participants in the symbolic dialogue, the focus must remain the patient's growth process.

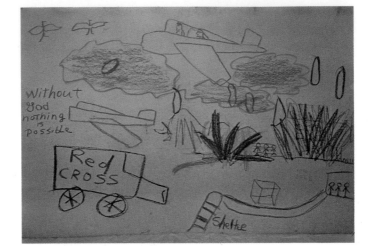

FIGURE 6.10: On the mural, the therapist visually explodes a bomb. This symbolic act releases feelings of destruction, rage and hostility which were contained and denied by the patients. Out in the open, this energy can be examined, directed and integrated.

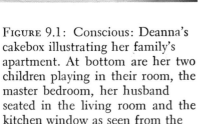

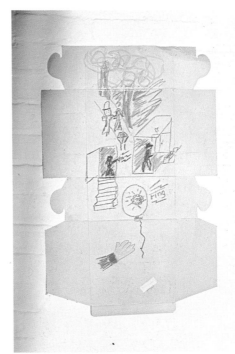

FIGURE 9.1: Conscious: Deanna's cakebox illustrating her family's apartment. At bottom are her two children playing in their room, the master bedroom, her husband seated in the living room and the kitchen window as seen from the street.

FIGURE 9.2: Unconscious: Deanna's initial dream in image form needs to be read from the bottom to the top. Her shadowy self representation appears walking arm in arm with the friendly policeman.

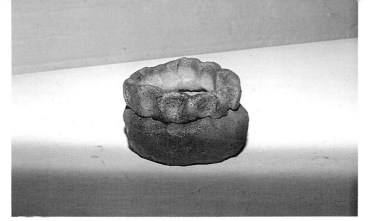

FIGURE 9.3: A first venture into a strange, new material and an exercise in centering produced the clay pinch pot with the pie crust rim.

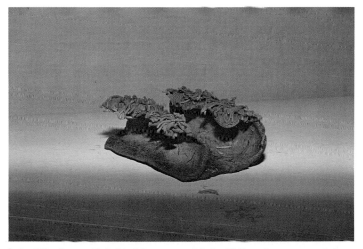

FIGURE 9.4: The beautiful double wave with bubbling foam revealed a split between a joyous freedom and an aching sadness.

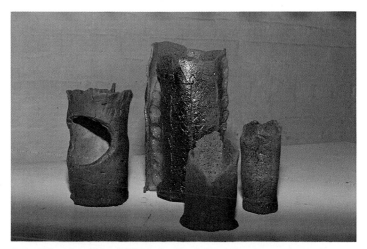

FIGURE 9.5: The family of hand built slab pots were never all attached as originally planned. The feminine/mother cylinder has a large opening suggesting both an openness and an emptiness.

F

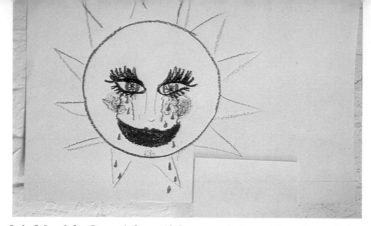

FIGURE 9.6: Mandala One: A beautiful, sunny lady smiling through her tears. D.'s polished persona belies her inner sadness and intimates an eventual rainbow.

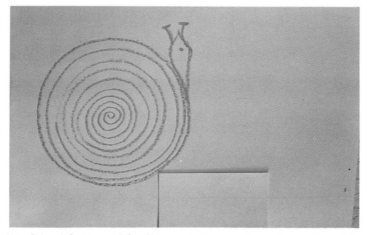

FIGURE 9.7: Mandala Two: The slow, spiraling snail so simply found her own way out of the tangled maze of the self. She is a monochromatic creature in lime green.

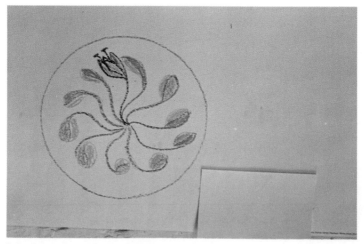

FIGURE 9.8: Mandala Three: While one young flower repeats the design of the snail's antennae, the other sprouts portend further growth.

G

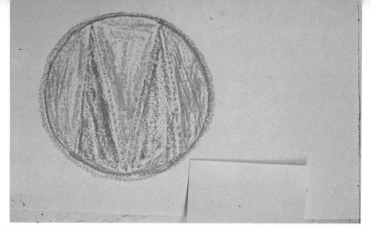

FIGURE 9.9: Mandala Four: The tension of opposites is expressed within the circle. Woman/Man, pink/green, yin/yang, valley/mountain are all drawn with great energy.

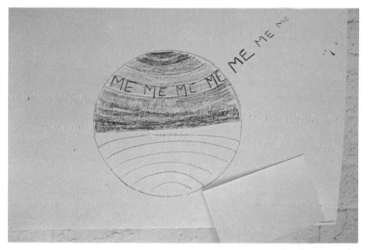

FIGURE 9.10: Mandala Five: D.'s rainbow of "ME" reveals the conscious self differentiated in many aspects with an equal area of unexplored territory "below" consciousness.

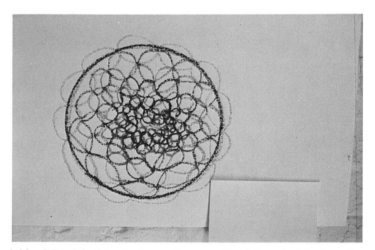

FIGURE 9.11: Mandala Six: A chrysanthemum in pink and red, the color of intense feeling, grew from a continuous line beginning at the center. The full bloom fulfills the promise of growth and integration in Mandala Three.

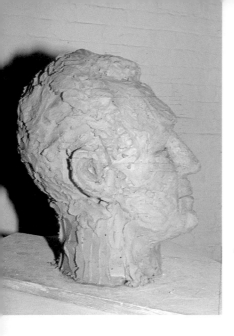

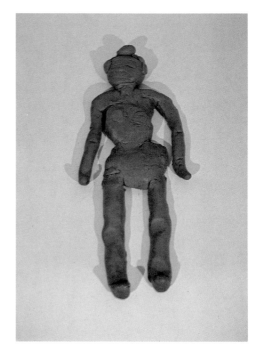

Figure 9.12: The sculptured clay head of D'.s father/animus/masculine element measures about 24" high and about 12" wide. The bust was eventually cast in plaster completing the creative process and achieving a significant therapeutic/life goal for Deanna.

Figure 14.1: Molding clay figures presented a means of working with Joanne on body image. This early figure in red plasticine of a woman was one of several figures which Joanne and I built together as part of the therapeutic/educative process.

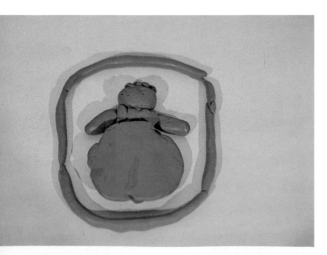

Figure 14.2: The last clay figure (in green plasticine) which Joanne produced, this figure of a baby girl, built without my assistance, expresses Joanne's emotional needs at this point in her treatment.

I. THEORY AND PRACTICE

1. Origins in Psychology

The neophyte art therapist would do well to study the origins and history of art therapy. Theory and practice have evolved from many crosscurrents which can be found in the fields of both psychotherapy and artistic creation. This chapter presents the psychological roots contributing to the evolution of art therapy; creativity theory roots appear later in the book. We are not attempting in this chapter to review all the literature. There are many books with which the student can become acquainted that offer a detailed, comprehensive survey, such as Hall and Lindzey's *Theories of Personality* (1). However, the reader will appreciate the following chapters if she has some sense of significant theories and forces in the area of human growth and development. Clearly, in psychotherapy as in art therapy, technique results from theory.

Within the area of therapeutic treatment by communication, there are three major schools of thought: psychodynamic determinism, humanistic psychology and behaviorism. Art has been integrated into each approach as a useful modality. But only in the last 30 years has art therapy grown into a profession in its own right. A delicate synthesis continues to take place between a psychological framework which articulates working theory and practice and our identification with the creative process on a personal level as working artists.

Psychodynamic

Any practitioner with a psychodynamic base owes a strong debt to Freud (2). His most important contribution was the refutation of rational materialism in the postulation of the unconscious, and belief in intrapsychic forces.

Within this conception, one of the most thorough and complex structures was laid for all future psychodynamic formulations. This structure postulates that man's psyche consists of conscious, pre-

3

conscious and unconscious levels of awareness. Primary thought process, originating in the unconscious, has its own separate energies and images. Freud's monumental opus, *The Interpretation of Dreams*, illustrates primary process at work. Through dream language, inner experiences, feelings and thoughts are expressed with their own unique logic. Our waking order of space and time does not apply. Secondary process refers to conscious awareness, logical thinking and deliberate symbol formation.

Freud presents the notion of the ego as a center, mediating and coping with outer and inner worlds. It responds to both primitive id forces and superego social controls. All three functions can operate with degrees of intensity at all levels of consciousness.

The acceptance of the irrational is necessary for the understanding of the whole reality of a person in most therapies, but particularly in art and creativity where spontaneity rules. Freud's postulation of a pre-conscious level of images just "below" awareness lays groundwork for the later development of Kris' (3) formulation of a psychology of creativity. As images function as connecting links among various levels of intrapsychic relatedness, artistic creation gives the individual the opportunity to harness the energies and images into a concrete manifestation.

Freud did ask patients to paint, particularly amorphous or diffuse dreams. Naumberg (4) further extends this point of view by developing a dynamic art therapy orientation which utilizes art as a medium to further therapeutic communication. Kramer (5), on the other hand, emphasizes the notion of sublimation, which has a psychoanalytic theoretical basis, and amalgamates the role of the artist and healer from a different point of departure. Art, in her view, offers a healing and binding quality to an individual who seeks a medium to capture forbidden impulses. We also owe to Freudian psychoanalysis the seminal contributions of dream theory, technique and interpretation, which are intimately connected to our understanding of the creative process.

Dream interpretation and free association were tools developed to explore the unconscious. Both contributed substantially to the evolution of art therapy technique. Freud saw psychoanalysis initially as a research tool, not as a treatment. The student entering this field would benefit from incorporating his essential attitudes of the unprejudiced, attentive listener.

Jung's (6) regard for imagination and creativity as a healing force stands as a cornerstone in the therapeutic dialogue. Jung further extended the role of the therapist as researcher-observer-listener to that of active participant. Perhaps less linear than free association, Jung's technique of active imagination encourages the patient to fantasize the continuation or possible conclusion of an ambiguous or interrupted dream situation. Feelings can be followed beyond words and manifested in painting, sculpture, and movement. Jung is most attractive to art therapy students for the importance he attributes to images. The psychic heritage of mankind, stored in the collective unconscious, passes in image from one generation to the next, unhampered by geographical or cultural boundaries.

An art therapist needs to recognize the language of imagery that is common to all; symbolic dialects differ from population to population. Jung saw the integration of opposites, on many levels, as the ongoing task of the individual throughout life. His therapeutic aim was one of individual growth, not "cure." Images expressed through art form a natural testing-ground for such "individuation."

Adler's (7) most appealing concept is that of the "creative self": Man continually creates his own personality. The administration of power and control of dynamic interpersonal forces by consciousness give meaning to life. Any art therapist who functions in an institution will find it useful to incorporate the Adlerian understanding of power! The order of birth is also seen as a social determinant of growth and development: The oldest, middle and youngest child each has a distinctly different experience of the world. The earliest recalled memory sometimes reveals a clue to one's lifelong psychological attitude. These concepts may be directly transposed into art therapy techniques that may give a clearer understanding of the patient's point of view.

The Neo-Freudians, such as Sullivan (8), Horney (9), and Fromm (10), help the art therapist gain a more sophisticated understanding of the subtleties of interpersonal operations. Object relations theory, (i.e. how one subjectively relates to the objective world), further extends this thesis and provides the useful notion of the transitional object. Winnicott (11) utilized art extensively in his work with children. The significance of the transitional object in establishing trust has become an invaluable concept, especially when we encounter narcissistic disorders.

Humanistic

Humanistic and object relations theories seem to naturally converge for the art therapist. The problem of existence is not adjusting oneself to the environment, but rather discovering the self emerging through a unique and individual process. This attitude also provides a working credo for the artist as well as the art therapist. Like Jung, Binswanger (12) saw the therapist and patient as partners in an attempt to discover how that process went astray, and how it might be more successfully adapted. Binswanger acknowledges the grounding of therapist and patient in humanity, relatedness and love. We see the soul of the art therapy process coming out of this movement. It is a less scientific and intellectual approach and is more "practical-livable." The real interpersonal relationship (an integral part of both object relations and humanistic schools) is of primary importance.

The art therapist aims for a difficult synthesis, integrating these notions with those of transference and resistance that will necessarily arise in the therapeutic relationship and in the art products.

Perls (13) is chiefly responsible for integrating a Freudian understanding of the structure of the psyche with Gestalt principles creating what we know as Gestalt therapy. Perls de-emphasizes early and final personality formation in the past and the repression of unpleasant experiences. Rather, he maintains a "here and now" attitude, giving an immediate, alive quality to the therapeutic encounter. Perls also draws heavily on Reich (14) in the notion of character armor: the creation of muscular tension-blocks in response to threatening situations. Gestalt art therapists borrow concepts from psychodrama (15), bioenergetics (16) and existential analysis (17). The "therapeutic act," which becomes an art in and of itself, seems to have some relevance. Thus, the impact of holding a hand or offering a creative gift to an emotionally impoverished patient may connote symbolic understanding on the deepest levels of communication. Gestalt art therapy attempts to combine creativity and nonverbal communication. Rhyme (18) and Rapp (19) are currently working with this approach and connect the joy of artistic expression with increased self-awareness.

Reik (20) contributes the concept of the third ear: The therapist utilizes her intuition to decipher undercurrents of meaning during the ongoing dialogue (similar to Ehrenzweig's (21) "unconscious scanning"). The use of the therapist's unconscious as an important basis for understanding the patient's communications enables the therapist to tap important inner resources. No ideal art therapy relationship could be complete without a central belief in the development of the self. Rogers (22) sets the stage in his client-centered therapy. This has further evolved into encounter and sensory awareness techniques. Maslow (23) also contributes to this movement with his emphasis on self-discovery and realization. The underlying threads of empathy, authenticity and affirmation of the worth of the patient are an intrinsic philosophical belief of any worthy therapeutic endeavor.

Behaviorism

Art therapists sometimes have difficulty utilizing the important tenets of behavior therapy (24). The techniques to modify the maladaptive stimulus-response pattern, e.g., operant conditioning, aversion conditioning and systematic desensitization can attain the therapeutic goals of increased functioning.

However, within the context of our understanding of art therapy, a classical behavior therapy approach is not an appropriate means of treating the whole person. Only if the art therapist broadens her understanding of all the complexities that surround human development can behavior modification techniques be best used to further individual coping. We must not allow "behaviorism" to read "conformity," interpreted as a threat to individuality. The research with autistic and mentally retarded children, as well as with a broad spectrum of neurotic disorders, substantiates claims to successful results. Art materials clearly provide the acute sensory stimulation (texture, color, odor) to implement conditioning techniques. For further elaboration of the use of behavior modification in art therapy, see Chapter 11 on Art Therapy in a School for Mentally Retarded Children.

As we review these three major schools of psychological thought, a fulcrum seems to emerge for the art therapist. By her training and discipline, symbolism becomes the means for creative and therapeutic development. Throughout the history of mankind, dreams, myths and folklore have always provided a source of communication and living wisdom.

As a result of Descartes' rational scheme of knowledge in the seventeenth century, our value system changed to one that worshipped the power of the word and logical, scientific thinking. Art emphasized external rather than internal realities. Dreams and mythic images became the forgotten language. As a result of the science of psychoanalysis, twentieth-century man has rediscovered the inner world.

The psychodynamic theory of symbolism gives us a basis to view man's secret wishes and fears; historical and cultural connections as viewed through archetypal images also come alive. Of late, ego psychologists find hidden coping mechanisms and possible solutions in fantasy or art production.

In the humanistic context, self-realization, as postulated by Maslow, becomes the right and goal of every human being. Maximizing one's self-growth potential includes expanding the boundaries of one's psychic consciousness. Energies and forces are neither denied nor repressed in the service of "adjustment." Included here is a greater awareness and respect for one's personal symbols, for they can be the medium for the discovery of the untapped self (25).

The art therapist is a specialist not only in a concrete symbolic language but also in other forms of nonverbal communication. In art therapy, symbols are found not merely in dreams and works of art, but can be lived out as a self-actualized form of identity. In fact, an authentic person must be in touch with his inner symbols, which are constantly being affirmed through creative, self-realizing acts. Complex sensory feeling experiences are locked into one's body and expressed in an entire style of life. One's life can be seen as a creative process or work of art. The art therapist is intimately involved in helping the individual harness symbolic manifestations into a meaningful form of existence.

The therapeutic act and the creative expression merge. As man becomes increasingly in touch with his symbols through any form of expression (art, dance, music, drama, poetry), we believe an increased sense of mastery develops. In order for symbols to be useful, they must be integrated into the self rather than flooding the boundaries of the ego in the service of expression.

Within this framework of humanistic and dynamic psychology, the art therapist can selectively apply the tools of behaviorism to strengthen and to further individual growth.

Listening on the most profound levels to human emotion, and using art as an arena to cope with existence and change maladaptive behavior patterns, the art therapist creatively synthesizes psychodynamic determinism and humanism. The enhancement of autonomy strivings we see in ego-psychoanalysis, the continual self-growth inherent in the individuation process, and the responsible, creative, loving self born of the existential experience converge to form our art therapy foundation. To the extent that a student can weave into a personal therapeutic matrix the various threads of her genesis and current individual growth process she will develop a creative, distinct professional style consistent with the best traditions of the artist.

Creativity is a further extension of the self-actualization process. It belongs to all rather than a few talented individuals. Art therapy, then, becomes open not only to a product orientation (which can be therapeutic), but also to a process deeply connected with self-expression and realization.

References

1. Hall, C. S. and Lindzey, G. *Theories of Personality*. New York: John Wiley and Sons, 1957.
2. Freud, S. *The Interpretation of Dreams*. Translated by Grill. New York: Modern Library, 1950.
3. Kris, E. *Psychoanalytic Explorations in Art*. New York: International Universities Press, 1952.
4. Naumburg, M. *Dynamically Oriented Art Therapy: Its Principles and Practices*. New York: Grune and Stratton, 1966.
5. Kramer, E. *Art Therapy in a Children's Community*. Springfield, Illinois: Charles C Thomas, 1958.
6. Jung, C. G. *The Portable Jung*. Ed. J. Campbell. Translated R. F. C. Hull. New York: The Viking Press, 1971.
7. Adler, A. *The Practice and Theory of Individual Psychology*. New York: Harcourt Brace, 1932.
8. Sullivan, H. S. *The Interpersonal Theory of Psychiatry*. 1st ed. New York: W. W. Norton, 1953.
9. Horney, K. *The Neurotic Personality of Our Time*. New York: W. W. Norton, 1937.
10. Fromm, E. *The Forgotten Language*. New York: Grove Press, 1951.
11. Winnicott, D. W. *Therapeutic Consultations in Child Psychiatry*. New York: Basic Books, 1971.
12. Binwanger, L. "Insanity as Life-Historical Phenomenon and as Mental Disease. The Case of Ilse." *Existence: A New Dimension in Psychiatry and Psychology*. Ed., R. May. New York: Basic Books, 1956.
13. Perls, F. S. *Gestalt Therapy Verbatim*. Lafayette, California: Real People Press, 1969.
14. Reich, W. *Character Analysis*. New York: Simon and Schuster, 1945.

15. Moreno, L. L. *Psychodrama and Group Psychodrama Monographs*. New York: Beacon House, 1946.
16. Lowen, A. *Language of the Body*. New York: Collier Books, 1958.
17. Wolstein, B. *Irrational Despair*. New York: Macmillan, 1962.
18. Rhyne, J. *The Gestalt Art Experience*. Monterey, California: Brooks/Cole, 1973.
19. Rapp, E. *The Creative Growth Experience*. New York: unpublished paper, 1971.
20. Reik, T. *Listening with the Third Ear*. New York: Pyramid Communications, 1948.
21. Ehrenzweig, A. *The Hidden Order of Art: A Study in the Psychology of Artistic Imagination*. Berkeley: University of California Press, 1967.
22. Rogers, C. *On Becoming a Person*. Boston: Houghton Mifflin, 1961.
23. Maslow, A. *Toward a Psychology of Being*. New York: Van Nostrand Reinhold, 1968.
24. Wolpe, J. and Lazarus, A. A. *Behavior Therapy Techniques*, New York: Pergamon Press, 1966.
25. Adler, G. *The Living Symbol: A Case Study in the Process of Individuation*. New York: Pantheon Books, 1961.

2. Becoming an Art Therapist

Defining the boundaries of art or therapy is an open invitation to get lost in a metaphorical muddle, conjuring up exquisite ambiguities. Nevertheless, the beginning student rightly demands clarification of a professional role model. Definitions are presented, cases are illustrated; yet an unsettled and anxious feeling often pervades the initial classes in art therapy. The interlocking processes of art, therapy, and personal development, the basic understructure of this field, are prodigious in scope and make enormous demands upon one's emotional and cognitive resources. Consequently, the sense of anxiety and excitement found during the introductory classes slowly transforms into waves of confusion and despair. Complex concepts and powerful affects emanating from patients, institutions and her own unresolved intrapsychic conflicts literally inundate the neophyte professional.

Learning art therapy demands a good deal of openness and self-confrontation. For many, this mode of learning is alien to their entire style of privacy and control. For many students, a respect for the right to withhold until they are ready to be more open is an absolute necessity if progress is to be made in this direction. The demand for openness can often be a strong conformity pressure that in and of itself needs some confrontation. Many a student will be able to receive support from peers and learn to counteract a sense of alienation as she shares strange and puzzling feelings. Even with this support, however, the art therapist soon finds personal therapy an absolute necessity and an aid in keeping an emotional hold on these difficult pressures. Defenses are constantly disrupted as the student becomes immersed in primitive impulses and imagos that erupt in the art therapy process. This constant preoccupation with the unconscious makes it virtually impossible for an intern to stand still in her own growth and expansion. This can be one of the most exciting parts of learning a new discipline. Hopefully, personal therapy will not be seen as a requirement but a challenge to enhance a sense of professional growth.

The issues discussed in this chapter can be best approached within

11

a supportive and enlightened supervisory relationship, which is an integral part of the learning experience whereby a student becomes a professional. An ongoing relationship exists between a student and an experienced practitioner of art therapy throughout the training period. Although there are many conceptions of supervision the kind of relationship consistent with the philosophy of this text deals with both the cognitive and the emotional development of a student. Thus, the art therapy supervisor is a resource person as well as someone who can subtly relate to the emotional issues that interfere with therapeutic effectiveness. A supervisor may also offer various art experiences that will stimulate the student's own creative development. Ideally, the student who maximizes supervision is the one who has enough ego strength to be open to and share with others her unconscious and also to hear and utilize available technical information.

The appropriate line between supervision and therapy may be unclear even to the most skillful supervisor. When complex resistances develop regarding problematic learning issues and the student's subjective experience outweighs her objective understanding, he may more effectively deal with these issues in personal therapy. Such resistance to taking a creative and autonomous stance to one's individual growth and learning can be seen in a number of ways, e.g., taking a passive, incorporative attitude towards the supervisor ("Tell me what to do, to say, to feel, etc.").

Each student intern requires an individual approach within the context of her characterological orientation. One may view supervision as a feeding, i.e., emotional nourishment that will ease the growth process. Another wants to use the power of the supervisor through submission and conquest. Still another may set up competitive situations and test out her mettle against the supposed superior authority. Fears regarding exposure often enter into the relationship and a need to be invulnerable may exist. The complexity of the attitudes seems as broad as any found in the therapeutic encounter. The underlying principle, therefore, is that each student attempts to utilize supervision to maximize her autonomous development. Her resistances to learning and changing are recognized and respected. A sense of support and nonjudgment would seem to be the ideal atmosphere for such a relationship to flourish. The student's goal in supervision is toward developing a personal therapeutic style consistent with her own growth rather than mimicking or idealizing a role model set forth by her supervisor. Without an effective and open dialogue with a supervisor, a student will be missing a most enriching part of his entire learning process.

Roughly speaking, problems in learning this difficult process can be broken down into two areas: 1) issues relating to the development of a professional role; and 2) the particular strengths and vulnerabilities an artist brings to a training program as she attempts to apply creativity to the interpersonal as well as the inanimate.

A constant refrain seems to resound through opening courses: "Who am I? What am I doing? Where am I going? How will this field make an effect on me?" Some students already have very definitive notions pertaining to these questions. Others seem completely lost and have but vague stirrings relating to these matters. Sooner or later, most students realize that ready-made definitions and roles are not appropriate or sufficient.

"What do I do with patients who only want to talk?" "Am I really doing art therapy when it sounds so much like psychotherapy?" "How about patients who like to dance or sing? Do they belong to another department?" "What if I am also drawn to these areas? Am I in the right program?" A developing art therapist may face these role dilemmas very early in her training. She receives little help from institutions or her professional elders in resolving these issues. Unfortunately, both parties may be much more comfortable with role definitions based on specified skills and functions.

The range of institutions where art therapy is practiced is broad; each setting presents a new set of opportunities and limitations. Superficially, art therapy can be practiced in so many different ways, it becomes difficult to comprehend a unifying concept. Art teacher, creativity specialist, social catalyst, psychotherapist: All seem to emerge and have special emphasis depending on the institution and/or the practitioner. Slowly, some students give up their quest for a role definition centered on skills or functions. Grudgingly for some, with relief for others, a process-oriented conception of art therapy develops. Creativity and therapeutic change become the internal anchor of a professional image. But this self-image does not appear without a good deal of soul-searching and anguish.

For those students who have not undergone personal therapy, the stirring-up of intrapsychic material caused by transferential or induced reactions can be a threatening experience. Some respond to this challenge and accept a new conception of a therapeutic process; the healer and the healed often exchange roles or occasionally provide a mutual function. An art therapy intern soon realizes the great similarities between the patient and herself. However, she is simultaneously expected to maintain boundaries and keep appropriate professional distance from the patient. The demands of this emotional balancing act are excruciating. A student responds at the deepest intrapsychic levels and must be able to separate these communications into the proper channels, i.e., induced reaction versus countertransference. Problems may be selectively shared with the patient. This juggling takes a tremendous amount of time and maturity before any professional works comfortably at so many levels. Old conceptions of humanism and authenticity are challenged. "How can I be responsive and caring and still give a patient room to grow and breathe?" When the complexities of this integration become too much to bear, the plea sounds once again: "What is an art therapist? Define the role so that I can avoid the pain of not knowing!"

In response to the ambiguities and complexities of a new learning situation, polarization of role models erupts. These conflicts often serve as resistances to learning; one easily becomes caught up in an endless dialogue that offers few creative answers to perplexing issues. The theoretical orientation of an intern may be either a strong art background or a strong psychology background. The resistances toward integration of an art experience approach with a more psychotherapeutic emphasis can be traced to the internal dynamics constellated within each person. Art for some has become a means of protection as well as an expression mediating the pressures of the inside and outside world. Explanations and psychological understanding are experienced as an intrusion. Art is an inexplicable and very private affair. Therapeutic implications of art are resented as they jar the student's personal homeostasis and manner of coping with threat. On the other hand, many trainees are drawn to the field of mental health as a means of gaining understanding of their own internal dynamics. Art therapy becomes an entrée into their own personal therapy. Frequently, this type of student feels compelled to have tight intellectual control over the learning process and wards off any breakthrough of spontaneous impulsive material that is part of a genuine art experience. The psychology-oriented student may well be more comfortable in approaching the creative process as a cognitive endeavor. For both the art-oriented student and the psychology-oriented student, a polarized debate as to the place of art in therapy avoids the integration that occurs through the joys of creativity and of self-discovery.

The person with an art education background brings to the therapeutic relationship a repertoire of projects that can be excellent vehicles for self-expression and development. These very same exercises can also be used as a means of avoiding the subtleties of interpersonal contact. Those who come from the field of occupational therapy may also be influenced by a task orientation. Perceptual retraining or socialization is overemphasized at the cost of an open, creative attitude and may well be a defensive maneuver to avoid overwhelming, alien and difficult feelings. Taking a step in the direction of having both patient and therapist discover the appropriate task or project makes the broad jump into creativity development.

In many settings, administrators have little conception of the scope of art therapy. Art therapists are seen as recreation workers, paraprofessionals, hybrid occupational therapists, or enlightened art teachers. As a consequence, the intern is constantly called upon to define her position and educate others. For many students, this is a very painful and endless struggle. At times, the intern is neglected and ignored. The young art therapist deals with fears of being assertive and aggressive in order to challenge preconceived notions and the political structure. She must also be sensitive to the institution's political undercurrents and not alienate herself from the working team. Many students do not want to be encumbered by these forces. They resent being part of a social matrix. Often the lament is heard, "Why can't I be left alone so I can do my thing?" Occasionally, deep transferences are acted out upon the institution, which only serves to make the student confused and ineffective.

A process definition of a professional role model is unacceptable in most institutions. This notion violates the pecking order and homeostasis of the prevailing structure. Psychiatrists, psychologists, and social workers often have short memories and forget their past battles to have an equal and expanding role on the mental health team. Now art therapists are forced to go through the same painful ordeal if they are to overcome a paraprofessional or technical image. To handle rage, withdrawal and acting-out and be able at the same time to communicate to one's peers and elders with a sense of dignity and forthrightness are tall orders for a novice professional.

An instructor who has the opportunity to teach both psychology and art students will be aware of some discernible differences between the two groups. Art students enter training programs with very special assets and liabilities. Although generalizations are difficult to make,

over the years, experienced faculty often are aware of broad trends
that demand recognition. Instructors would do well to avoid the
error of relating to artists solely as psychological trainees.

The prototypical art-oriented student is full of inconsistencies and
paradoxes. Wary of the obvious, suspicious of anything that smacks
of the manipulative, art has often been a means to channel a distinct
sense of individuality; for others, it has been a means of survival. Now
outspoken and nonconforming, now insulated and private, an artist
searches for contact and relatedness. Education programs in the past
have proved a dreary disappointment. Many hope art therapy will
provide an answer for the channeling of original expression within the
human and social context. Action-oriented and often impulsive, theory
gets in their way. Many are more than willing to risk leaps into the
unknown if only to find meaning and significance in their work. Soon,
massive doses of affects emanating from the work shake the very
underpinnings of their psychic foundations. Loneliness and depression
that have been masked through art and symbolism break through into
consciousness. Many wonder if they have gotten much more than they
bargained for. The following comments attempt to highlight some of
these growing pains and critical issues the typical artist encounters
in a training program.

If students come to a new program frustrated in their ability to find
their own creative energy, they may hope that art therapy will give
them answers to their own creative blocks. These fears are often exhibited in the manner in which a trainee approaches her patient. Some
students are frightened of a patient's losing control because of their
own internal anxieties: She subtly sabotages any attempt by the
patient to loosen up by the use of structured materials and by being
overly interpretive. Another, because of her own inner problems'
regarding structure and limits, finds it difficult to transmit an inner
sense of discipline. Students' fear of the cognitive area ultimately has
its genesis in dependency, power and hostility; however, many do
not see the connection between their resistances toward cognitive
material and their personal anxieties in helping patients deal with
structure and reality. This dissociation between a student's academic
and professional life is a manifestation of a splitting process that makes
learning and change so difficult.

A common controversy in the field centers in the area of aesthetic
judgment. Those who have strong investments in the field of art
experience a basic violation when standards of aesthetics are abused.

Others view this approach as overly judgmental and feel it restricts the entire flow of communication. "Standards" sound very close to "conformity," which has been the stimulus for a long-standing rebellion. Distance from such a personalized point of view on the part of all concerned is needed. Everything expressive is not always beautiful and deserving of praise. For the therapist to help patients harness, cope, and crystallize their feelings and imagery through a cohesive representation of art may offer a new feeling of mastery. On the other hand, those trainees who insist on certain preconceived standards at the cost of freedom and spontaneity may well look to the areas of power and control filtering into their therapeutic attitudes.

Exhibitionism in the arts, when truly expressive and integrated, can be a positive avenue of self-affirmation. However, this impulse may be dissociatively acted out with patients and materials. Often, too, the art therapist plays the game of show and tell with her patient's art products. A therapist's power cannot arise from the display of her patient's paintings as a means of covering some of her own inner sense of impotence.

Another caution for artistic expression lies in the area of touch and sensuality. Art therapists often express unsatisfied needs for touch and intimacy that are not sublimated through normal interpersonal experiences. This delicate balance can be upset easily as patients and materials interact, causing a good deal of tactile excitement. For many, this is a positive experience. For others, however, erotic stimulation can overpower both participants in the dialogue, causing a flooding of the student's ego. The understanding of the principles of timing and rhythm is difficult to apply judiciously when the therapist's need for contact interferes with good judgment.

Many young trainees are both fascinated and trapped by their patients' unconscious communications. Not all symbolic communications connect with a quest for identity. Some material is discursive in nature and meant to be an avoidance of the reality problems of existence. Art therapists, if they themselves are lost in fantasy, may be unable to make this distinction.

Art therapists are constantly flooded by induced reactions ignited by the patient and the art process. Rage, intense eroticism, and anxiety of panic proportions are but a few of the internal vibrations that resonate in a therapeutic relationship. In the past, the art work of the artist has been a safe insulation and shock absorber from difficult affects that must now be dealt with in a more direct manner. The art therapist must constantly be aware of subtle maneuvers to avoid direct expression, which requires the development of an observing ego that listens and discriminates among many levels of communication. This observing ego aids the therapist in taking a more objective view of a subjective experience. Also involved in this process is the development of a concerned empathy, to be differentiated from sympathy. Placating patients by inundating them with gifts or approval may be one way to deaden or avoid rage, while hostility and curtness, as well as the use of certain aggressive materials, may cover the warm, sensitive parts of an interaction.

Art therapists need to be encouraged to accept a wide range of feelings as part of a normal therapeutic engagement. Difficulties in dealing with certain affects can be observed through a tendency to repress, dissociate or overemphasize certain aspects of communication. Discriminations between rage, vindictiveness, sadism, spite, and indignation can all be jumbled and lack specificity when one is under fire. Ultimately, all these feelings can be used as positive means to effect change. Thus, for example, the therapist's perception of her own indignation can be used as an important learning tool, particularly with patients who have lost their will to fight back.

A central issue for the art therapist is the distinction among separation, loneliness and solitude. Occasionally the artist has been lonely as well as alone during major parts of her life. Art has been a companion and has partially allayed a sense of emptiness. Often there are deep scars in these areas which become stirred up as she faces her patients' feelings of loss and abandonment. Her identification with the lost child in the patient makes the drawing of clear boundaries between therapist and patient a difficult task. Under the guise of being humanitarian, a therapist can lose her sense of self and become hopelessly lost in over-identification with the patient's grief and loneliness. A significant jump in learning is made by the student who realizes that she does not necessarily desert a patient when she goes home at night.

Separation, abandonment, and helplessness constantly surround the budding art therapist. Not to push the patient while experiencing his extreme pain will take a lot of discipline. To feel the desperate rage of a depression without attempting to manipulate superficial change virtually puts one through a wringer. Some depressed patients do need concrete help; others simply require the presence of the therapist. The art therapist diagnostically discerns these differences and uses materials, as well as feelings, in response to this discrimination. Those therapists who have unresolved problems regarding mothering will find it a difficult task to distinguish in the patient feelings of emptiness that arise from fears of intrusion, as contrasted to emotional impoverishment. Feeding and caring cannot be the magic solution to all of life's problems.

Involved in all the issues regarding growth is a gradual transition from simultaneous helplessness and seeming omnipotence to a professional autonomy that is purposeful, free, and yet controlled; the cognitive part of the therapist is integrated into a real sense of knowing. The omnipotence utilized as part of the creative process now rests more comfortably with a more authentic sense of power. Grandiosity is now used as a constructive therapeutic force which allows the therapist to take chances, reach into the unknown, and breech new frontiers. At the same time she can laugh at herself, forgive her errors, and recognize that her wish to play God must exist side by side with her own frail humanity. This degree of self-confidence and ease comes with years of struggle and only after a good deal of stumbling.

The every essence of the artistic experience negates authority. The negation is both the strength and the weakness of the artist. Many interns become threatened when faced with the need to set boundaries and limitations. Gradually they recognize an inner sense of authority comes from competence and knowledge rather than power. Some find this a rather difficult transition and tend to subtly stimulate the patient's own rebellion and loss of inner structure. A few may become power-oriented in their approach to patients. In spite of these problems, the individualistic nature of an artist may be the very answer to a patient's hungry need for identification with a model who refuses to submit to society's madness. If anything, the artist may be uniquely qualified to comprehend the sanity of a "disturbed" patient.

The art therapist brings with her the child who has found beauty, exploration and the wonder of discovery. Play, when used in the service of creativity, is an inherent part of the art therapy process. It is also a unique talent of the artist who, hopefully, will not forget this strength when she attempts to grow and mature in other areas of life. The art therapist who moves from the adult to the child and back again may be able to make that unique synthesis of discipline, freedom, and excitement and apply it to her therapeutic relationships. In technical terms, an observing ego, free and autonomous, allows the unconscious room to explore, discover and mold new solutions to old problems.

Becoming an art therapist is a rigorous and demanding course of self-development. There is room along this path for regression, depression and reevaluation. So-called mistakes, as in any art—or life—endeavor, can be transformed into new solutions and learning experiences. With this in mind, an art therapist may slowly begin to meet the complex challenges of her professional assignments and to experience the joy and satisfaction of growth in the therapeutic relationship.

3. Theoretical Perspectives

The art therapist travels within two worlds. The inner sphere contains the power of a unifying art experience—the regeneration required to rediscover a centeredness or internal rhythm of being. Through the art experience a worn and tattered self comes together and mends. At the same time, the art therapist recognizes the importance of an outside world. There are people and objects to see, to hear, and to touch. Messages seek receptors; social acts validate and confirm the self. Without this interactive process, survival becomes painful and nearly impossible. Discipline, control and the building of skills to communicate and cope with the outside are necessities.

To fulfill the dual conditions of such a venture, the art therapist induces a non-goal-oriented, holistic, and non-rational mode of functioning in his work. A surge of energy takes over one's very being as one lets go or loses control allowing the creative rebirth experience. For many, this aspect of art therapy makes a primary contribution to a resolution of life issues. At the same time, the art therapist also mediates a flow from an internal rhythm discovered through the art with a flood of confusing external stimuli. As with much art work, the art therapist travels simultaneously on different levels of consciousness. At the deepest plain there is a symbolic connection that feels like a deep drinking in of one's very essence. On another level, an observing, evaluating, synthesizing ego makes some sense and order out of our preconscious and unconscious stirrings. Depending on a whole set of factors, a focus or point of direction is taken by the therapist that expedites a life-giving process. This complicated back and forth negotiation evolves with difficulty. Art therapy has something very basic and viable to offer in facilitating this synthesis. In order to move toward this complicated integration, the art therapist develops a fluid theoretical model that evolves within each clinical situation. The subtle textures of relatedness, the range of emotional coloration coming from the dialogue, the balance of transference versus the real relationship, plus the internal and external compositions, constantly challenge the therapist's inventiveness.

Art therapists use their creativity to discover the theory that blends these forces together. Heavy theoretical investments in a particular point of view only serve to disconnect the therapist from using himself in this manner. Ideally, an art therapist identifies with creation, process, and change. He is equally cognizant of the importance of being, connection, and self-realization (1). These are the principles for an art therapy journey. Theory and techniques are less formidable issues as the practitioner becomes more sophisticated in assessing and relating the personality dynamics of each individual situation. For example, some patients require the broadening of their perceptual horizons. Others may need a cognitive sense of their feelings. For many, a cathartic release of repressed affects revitalizes the entire personality. Some have a painful need to get in touch with a centered-ness lost through life experience. Dosage, timing, and responsiveness all contribute to an art therapeutic approach. Theory is not an answer or solution for the anxiety of not knowing. The courage to wait, to experience, to discover the theory that fits the particular therapeutic encounter would seem a mark of the creative art therapist. Placing patients into a ready-made theoretical framework interferes with the capacity to see, to hear, and to respond with an authentic freshness. Theoretical conceptions, in fact, emanate from experiences, deriving from emotional encounters rather than a preconceived intellectualized map, and becoming an integral part of the therapist's perception. Readings, case discussions, and lectures provide helpful stimulation. However, when the therapist faces the patient, this knowledge, if it has had real impact upon the practitioner, will spontaneously arise and be utilized in the flow of therapeutic communication.

Varying theoretical orientations and related techniques lend them-selves to the employment of different personal resources by the art therapist. For example, one can envision a long-term therapeutic relationship which takes years to evolve to a point of reconstructive reorganization of the patient's personality (2). The patient perhaps is frightened of closeness and may require a slow building of trust. In such cases, the therapist waits, listens, and is attentive as he slowly perceives the images of the past and present as they synthesize and surface into consciousness. To an outside observer, nothing seems to have happened. Yet a slow building is going on. The therapist develops tolerance and discipline that constantly relate to the ebb and flow of these undercurrents. For some, this slow process may put too high a demand on the capacity to wait and listen without ostensible results.

By contrast, a workshop leader invited to visit a college campus is requested to give a one-session demonstration of the inherent possibilities available in using art therapy techniques (3). The situation calls for an action-oriented, emotionally reactive and self-assertive personality who can introduce a good deal of drama into the workshop. The therapist is both actor and theater director while the classroom becomes a stage. The theory that develops in the clinical situation, as in the college setting, arises out of the express needs of the therapeutic encounter. Ideally, the exposition of the clinical details will help reveal the method of communication.

Patients have different capacities to experience and understand themselves. For some, relationships and experiences are viewed as mirror reflections of their internal constellation. The therapist, in understanding these particular dynamics, will use his technique and knowledge of object relation theory (4) as a positive force to aid individuals in growing. Therapists heavily invested in a professional image directed towards giving interpretations may not hear the real growth needs of narcissistic individuals. To recognize the distinction between an object and a narcissistic transference makes all the difference in the development of an art therapeutic relationship. The patient's art work can become a transitional object which starts the process of externalization of toxic introjects. On the other hand, it can become a vehicle through which he receives timely interpretations when the therapeutic process becomes encumbered in resistances. In the latter instance, the patient is displaying enough of a cooperative and free ego to experience this approach as helpful (object transference). In the former, an interpretative approach would be felt as an assault by the therapist (narcissistic tranference). An art therapist discerns these differences and responds with the appropriate therapeutic act.

Rogerian techniques have been successfully utilized with patient populations with relatively strong and intact egos (5). Adolescents, for instance, can often benefit from self-disclosure given a fairly permissive and open climate. Children, likewise, who have strong developmental needs to grow and integrate, find this approach unifying. As patients become embedded in pathology and passive, sticky resistances to change appear, the therapist can integrate a Rogerian philosophy with techniques that deal with negativism and firm defenses. The concept of resistance does not exist in non-directive therapy. However, the negative, walled-off and self-defeating patient rarely works well within a permissive, accepting atmosphere. Thus, to discover the appropriate means to overcome internalized characterological resistances becomes a creative extension of the art therapist. To cite an example, the passive-aggressive personality will forget, deny, and literally display clear evidence of his hostility all over the therapy room. The creative art therapist innovates methods that break through this patient's armor by mirroring his behavior. Insisting on a "therapeutic art experience" for this type of patient who employs art as part of a contempt system is not constructive. To conclude that he cannot make use of art therapy limits and restricts the art therapist's role unnecessarily. The requirements of the clinical situation, as well as the skills of a particular practitioner, determine the boundaries of a professional role.

Autistic children offer an excellent illustration of this point (6). Their world contains frightening, shattering and disconnected perceptions, partial imagos and disorganizing affects. The art therapist introduces a symbiotic relatedness and a building of a body ego through tracing, touch, and other sensory techniques. Feelings need concretization and adaptive patterns require reinforcement. The art therapist's role in accomplishing these goals necessitates a very high order of training and competence. Because of the very specialized background of the artist in sensory modalities, clinical and artistic skills can merge to create a very valuable practitioner who is ideally suited to meet the demands of these particular children.

Some may wonder if this point of view obscures the difference between an art therapist and a psychotherapist. In actual practice, there may be very little difference. Is there a justification for a separate field of art therapy? Perhaps, for the field of psychotherapy cuts across many different professional lines: Psychotherapy is not the separate province of psychiatry, social work or psychology. Today, under more enlightened clinical administrations, all members of a team ranging from the ward attendant, nurse, or psychiatrist, perform therapeutic work. Each professional, because of his formal training, brings something special and characteristic to the treatment process. The psychologist may bring an emphasis on the scientific and experimental, while the psychiatrist has as a special forte the biological and clinical pathology. So, likewise, the artist contributes his knowledge of the creative process. An art therapist is well qualified to help patients make the difficult integration because of his understanding of the interplay of creativity development and a psychotherapeutic approach.

The artist has often captured through his work the essence of human existence: the pain of being, the fear and need of love, the beauty and despair of mankind. Likewise, the art therapist gravitates towards a very humanistic and responsive type of therapy that expresses this heritage.

Psychoanalytic theory and understanding does not necessarily mean an intellectualized or dehumanized approach to one's work. Thus, the art therapist who offers a "messy art experience" to a tightly controlled and rigid patient may make a significant statement of cognition. This statement is based on a sensitive understanding and need not always translate itself into a direct verbal interpretation. The above implies that human relatedness and responsiveness are more important than a particular orientation. Likewise, humanness belongs to no one particular school of thought.

The rather hollow arguments of the "here and now" versus the genetic approach often reach the point of polarization. Good treatment, regardless of orientation, is alive and dynamic. Past may be lived in the present as well as re-experienced in the reconstruction of the past. At the same time, an art therapist will find it helpful to know when a preoccupation with the present avoids painful past affects. On the other hand, it is also a commonplace occurrence for a preoccupation and a concern with the past to avoid the present. With each patient, the therapist explores and discovers the apex of emotional cathexis and follows a particular journey with this as his guideline.

Along the same vein, the art therapist's accessibility to such concepts as object relations, character structure, and transference does not preclude a humanistic interchange. As the therapist becomes less threatened by the onslaught of projections and forces within himself, he also acts as a model for relearning by the patient. Some patients literally hunger for internalizations. Others need someone who can relate and respond in a sensitive manner. Many patients do not require "cure" as much as the warmth and responsiveness of another. The art therapist who can truly see, hear, and communicate may touch a self literally starved for relatedness. This is particularly true for some depressive patients who require a transitional object for growth. Art therapy would seem especially applicable in these instances. The nonverbal quality of the interchange has all the ingredients of an early primary relationship, especially important and relevant in working through a depressive problem. The tactile quality, in fact, can be a means for making new internalizations crucial in repairing a symbiotic disturbance.

Regardless of the theoretical bias of the practitioner, symbolic expression characterizes the language of the therapeutic dialogue. In some instances, when the patient does not have the tools to visualize images, the art therapist may stimulate symbolic play as an educational experience. For example, a therapist can introduce mandalas to a patient as a tool for self-representation. Patients need to touch and experience their personal symbols to further the identification process. Needless to say, a political or intellectual indoctrination of symbolic meanings through constant interpretations may well disconnect rather than integrate an inner life.

Theory and practice cannot be discussed in a social vacuum. Patient populations vary widely from institution to institution. For instance, art therapists increasingly work in rehabilitation centers, where a common goal is to move post-hospitalized psychiatric patients back into the mainstream of society in a relatively short period of time. The art therapist, by necessity, develops a profound knowledge of ego psychology to function effectively as a member of rehabilitation team. Social and vocational functioning provides an important focus for the art therapy experience, in which the patient builds ego strength. Frustration tolerance, time perspective, reality testing and judgment —to name a few—are intensely observed and reconstructed within an art therapy situation. Art may still have the same dynamic meaning as in childhood—to play as well as test oneself and build a feeling of competence. An art therapist working in a rehabilitation center will need a sensitive understanding of materials and the psychic demands they produce on patients (see Chapter 16 on Art Materials). In addition, the discussion emanating from the interaction of an art group provides a fertile ground to explore and understand one's social functioning within a safe and supportive climate. Obviously, transference and characterological differences occur and need attention. Although limited time with the post-hospitalized patient may prevent the working-through of all reconstructive problems, there often exists enough autonomy of ego functions to permit alteration and change even if there is limited reorganization of intrapsychic process.

By contrast, an art therapist may function in a hospital setting

where the goals of treatment are long range and intensive. Primitiviza-
tion and regression of ego functioning characterize the hospital patient
population. In selected cases, a psychoanalytic approach may be
necessary, entailing a profound knowledge of pregenital and symbiotic
communications and the use of art therapy techniques that facilitate
such a slow reorganization (see also Chapter 6, Imagery: Part II).
The therapist, cognizant of both inner and outer pressures on the
patient, moves from the symbolic to the concrete, from the unconscious to the conscious, and attempts to build an ego by channeling
frightening affects into images. He also provides an atmosphere that
will enhance communication, specificity and connection.

From another perspective, art therapists now find openings in
educational systems (7). The art educator-therapist may, more often
than not, work with normal populations. Rarely will he have the
time to spend with individual cases, and the art product may have
some partial importance in terms of the aims and conditions of the
institution. The art therapist's knowledge of psychology and creativity
must be synchronized with educational goals. In addition, art can
be used as a means of both expressing creative energy and offering a
climate to neutralize inner conflicts. Interpretive therapeutic approaches have limited usefulness in these settings. Play and activity
group techniques provide excellent vehicles for dramatic interchange
and study of the child's life situation. Problems may arise regarding
a conflict of therapeutic and educational goals as the classroom
structure has its inherent conditions and limitations. However, the
art therapist will accomplish a good deal by recognizing emotional
communication even if there is some partial lid on full cathartic expression. Increasingly, art therapy as practiced in a school combines
with remedial tutoring. It has been hypothesized that the sensory,
imaginative, and conceptual factors of a learning situation interplay
and create an important developmental experience for reading. Many
students, without the sensory or imaginative experience, may well
encounter extreme difficulty in learning to read. The compartmentali-
zation of art and creativity from other significant parts of the cur-
riculum paints a dull world where learning is neither fun nor connected to any internal process. Abstract academic material becomes
more comprehensible and concrete when visualized through art work.
Gradually, educators are beginning to realize the importance of
creativity development not as a frill but as an important aspect of a
total process in learning.

Hopefully, the art therapist employs his creativity to participate in any number of situations so his talents and assets are maximized. In each area, he evaluates the developmental needs necessary to carry on a growth process and provides the creative means to release energy and growth. During the course of treatment, the needs of patients change and require a constant re-evaluation and reorganization of theoretical terms and implementations. Broadly speaking, patients may need building or uncovering or perhaps a combination of both. For many, especially for geriatric patients, the art therapy experience helps to pull life experiences together. In other instances, it facilitates the working-through of body trauma and separation, as on the pediatrics unit. The art therapist is not bound by a set of duties, functions, or materials. He perceives what each therapeutic situation offers, and fluidly moves in so he can use himself in the most creative and effective manner.

The theoretical and practical demands made upon the art therapist are enormous. Comparisons can be easily drawn with the discipline and demand of becoming a fine artist, which involves a lifetime of learning and change. Techniques and theories develop from a personal order. The work of the artist, as well as of the art therapist, has a very organic quality connecting to his style of life. In its fullest sense art therapy synthesizes personal, emotional and cognitive growth, and as this integration evolves a unique practitioner arrives on the scene whose art and creativity bring a very special dimension to the process of unifying the individual and enhancing therapeutic change.

References

1. Maslow, A. *Creative Attitude*. New York: Psychosynthesis Research Foundation, 1963.
2. Sechehaye, M. A. *Symbolic Realization*. New York: International Universities Press, 1960.
3. See case study by Susan E. Gonick-Barris, Chapter 15.
4. Jacobson, E. *The Self and the Object World*. New York: International Universities Press, 1964.
5. Rogers, C. *On Becoming a Person*. Boston: Houghton Mifflin, 1961.
6. See case study by Susan Mann, Chapter 12.
7. Pine, S. "Fostering Growth Through Art Education, Art Therapy and Art in Psychotherapy." *American Journal of Art Therapy*. Vol. 13, No. 2, Jan. 1974.

4. Creativity Development

A solid theoretical foundation in creativity development is critical for the aspiring art therapy student. This knowledge, combined with skills in therapeutic change, places the practitioner in a unique position in the field of mental health.

The purpose of this chapter is to synthesize psychoanalytic knowledge with techniques and functions that stimulate creativity development. There are some crucial studies in analytic literature that provide an appropriate point of departure.

Ernst Kris views the study of art as part of the study of communication (1). Within this context, the process of artistic creation is broken down into three distinct spheres: There is a sender, a receiver, and a message. The message, or the work of art, is in part similar to a dream. One sees a multifaceted integration on a variety of psychic levels and structures manifested through an interplay of visual imagery. This message is an invitation to a common experience in the mind, to an experience between artist and audience as they discover new depths of meaning to the world.

Kris draws our attention to the ego of the artist. The expression of regression in the service of the ego, with the concomitant implications of allowing fantasies to flood one's being in order to regain mastery, brings a crucial aspect of artistic creation into focus. The essence of his thesis is the regulation of the ego and the individual's ability to bind, neutralize and channel energy toward creative work. Yet this description often leaves much to be desired. Perhaps more accurately, we are dealing with a different orientation of life, with attitudes, values, and responses divergent from a Western point of view. Central to a creative orientation, therefore, may be a shift to a nonrational, paradoxical, ambiguous state of experience from a rational, goal-oriented approach. Associated with this shift, the individual seems to be gripped by introjects that have confluent ego

This chapter appeared in its original form in *Art Psychotherapy*: *An International Journal*, Vol. 1, Number 2, Fall 1973. Pergamon Press, New York.

functions and energies. These intrapsychic forces can shake the essence
of a human being (2). If these energies are neutralized, they have the
ability to stimulate and intensify communication on a primary level.

Any study of creative ability must include the whole area of nonverbal communication. Renee Spitz, a psychoanalytic researcher in
child development, refers to this primary relationship as co-anesthetic
organization (3). To quote Spitz, "Here sensing is extensive, primarily
visceral, centered in the automatic nervous system and manifests
itself in the form of emotions." Adults, he states, who have retained
the capacity to make use of one or several of these categories of
perception and communication, belong to the exceptionally gifted.
But, as Noyd, another psychoanalytic theoretician points out, primary
communication is mutual (4). Hence, the specific pattern, he states,
of communication characteristic of early mother-child dyads is mod-
eled on a combination of two factors: those contributed by the mother
and those inherent in the infant. Thus, the primary mode of communication between mother and child can be one of looking, touching, and/or cooing. This behavior can be observed in a wide variety
of relationships. The capacity, however, to relate to these very sub-
liminal cues both from within and without may be the source of the
artist's ability to see, hear, and experience the world with a sense of
freshness and originality. A highly developed sense of nonverbal communication enhances his ability to break through the often stereotyped
barriers of verbal communication.

Essential to this primary mode of communication is the artist's
belief and trust in his work. These qualities can be found in the artist's
friendship, marriage and therapy relationships.

Psychological research in the area of creativity has been growing.
Some of the most important work emanates from the University of
California where Barron has spent a considerable amount of time
studying various groups of artists (5). The conclusions culled from
his studies point to three major factors connected with creativity:
1) The artist seems concerned with complexity rather than simplicity;
2) the artist seems to be more open perceptually and resistant to
premature closure; 3) the artist often relies on his intuitive abilities.
The implications of this research are provoking. Hopefully, the well
trained art therapist will avoid the pitfalls of seeking simple solutions
for complex problems. He will also need the courage to wait and listen
and avoid inappropriate solutions. The creative therapist must also
address himself to the uncomfortable issue of premature closure with

its concomitant feelings of anxiety and ambiguity. Finally, he must employ his creativity to create environments conducive to the enhancement of intuitive and/or nonverbal communication. This environment or atmosphere would allow the therapist to replicate, for therapeutic purposes, a multitude of mother-child dyads, and relate to the specific imagery this relationship brings forth. As a specialist in nonverbal communication, he develops the capacity to empathize and to resonate with the patient. He mirrors, responds pictorially, and communicates graphically a whole range of textural messages. The art therapist has an empathetic ability to ebb and flow with the many waves of psychic expression generic to this process. At times, he may function as an ego support in order to set the stage for the release of neutralized energy, associated with primary introjects which have been externalized through the power of the creative relationship.

An art therapy relationship may seem strangely close to a love affair. This love affair may have some of the ingredients of a touching sweetness, or a sublime blissfulness. It contains all the trusting qualities of an early mother-child relationship where the basic mode of communication is one of a soft touch or perhaps a sweet sound. The therapist's response may be a reflection or a partial glimmer that is rarely verbally recognized. The words used would be graphic if not poetic. Object relatedness is often secondary, since premature emphasis on object relatedness may interfere with the creation of this generative partnership. The art therapist watches closely in order to respect the delicate movement along the closeness-distance continuum. Thus, as the creative dialogue charters itself in the most primitive layers of psychic organization, the early fears of being swallowed, abandoned, or annihilated can be mobilized easily. On the instinctual layer of a creative operation, strong cannibalistic urges are sometimes neutralized. The patient often needs the space to constructively use this energy to capture and to swallow his world, if only to send it forth with new meaning. For many, too great a closeness overwhelms the ego in its struggle for mastery or control. Yet, somewhere in the background, with this undercurrent of relatedness he may have the courage to brave the isolation of being with himself and to work towards creating an authentic statement.

As the art therapy relationship is fostered, a touching adoration can develop. On other occasions, the narcissistic investment and omnipotence remain largely within the patient as his work becomes literally a highly cathected appendage of himself.

Likewise, the therapist ultimately may become an appendage. To determine the locus of the narcissistic investment is of prime importance in assessing the appropriate form of relatedness. On the level where the therapist is but an appendage, his ability to accept this role with minimal interference may be a condition in the determination of his effectiveness. Many a therapist cannot bear such an insignificant position and experiences a degree of narcissistic injury.

Where the investment is within the relationship rather than the work, the omnipotence of a therapist, as manifested by a glowing adoration by the patient, must be accepted with a minimum of counterdefensive maneuvers. For some, this can be experienced as a great burden. However, the art therapist can effectively use this relationship as a source of stimulation and encouragement. The identification process, which may be introjective, is in and of itself not necessarily destructive. The determining factor will be the quality of the identification: Does it function as a bridge to further autonomy or does it lead to a sterile imitation of the therapist?

The creative process contains magical and omnipotent forces that serve both as a basis for keenly accurate perceptions and as a source of primitive fear and retaliation. The patient may need a good deal of support in his challenge to the world as he occasionally displays a grandiose flourish and abandon in his work. Yet, as he encounters approbation rather than punishment, the release of tension may well serve as the basis for motivation to delve deeper in exploration and discovery.

Security is not always possible when there is a bombardment of stimuli on a patient's ego that is already fragmented and disconnected. At times, a subtle restriction of stimuli may well give him the required protection. In contrast, others who are overly tight and rigid may need a certain degree of freedom and stimulation to loosen up the controls. Occasionally, music in the background seems to break through the defenses and allow the connection to be made in the preconscious. On other occasions, the use of surprise or shock can have a catalytic effect.

The vulnerability to narcissistic injury can never be underestimated when one deals with the creative process. As a patient displays to the world part of his most primitive, naked self, direct and frontal confrontation can be experienced as an assault that does nothing but raise defenses and lower the communication in the creative dialogue. One may wonder, therefore—if one cannot criticize—how the whole process of working through an integration takes place. To point out various avenues of exploration rather than to deal with the limitations of a work is a notion that every good teacher has in his professional equipment. To build rather than to tear down seems too obvious even to mention. Yet, all too often, one hears the mutilated accounts of aspiring artists, shattered from their learning experience rather than reinforced in their conviction that they dare to be what they are.

Basically, the art therapist must be as in tune with an individual's ego resources as with the underlying layer of preconscious fantasy. To assess when a person's ego integrative capacity has received maximum taxation or when he needs encouragement to remain in the field of battle is not always an easy chore.

The act of forcing more control may increase resistance to the flow of preconscious materials. To learn how not to push, to let things grow, to be able to know when to walk away, to be able—once you have the inspiration—to build rather than to jump from one thing to another are all ego techniques that the art therapist must have at his disposal. At times, there is too early a closure. Perhaps the anxiety accompanying the lack of closure pushes the individual towards over-simplification. Together, through a mutual identification, patient and therapist must face the paradoxes and inconsistencies and allow them to germinate until a more complete unity occurs.

Involved in the authentic relationship is the ability of the art therapist to distinguish what is truly artistic and creative. To discern the work that can stand alone, as contrasted to material that is in the service of exhibitionism or rebellion, is another important task of the therapist. As the therapist responds according to what is truly authentic, he may also help the patient perceive what is honest and direct.

On occasion, the patient may have difficulty in going on and challenging new and different areas of exploration. It is up to the art therapist to observe and deal with this occurrence, for often there is a fear of letting go and dipping once again into the preconscious layer.

The sense of touch pervades all areas of artistic integration. One of the most sensitive issues, however, is the actual physical "laying of hands" on the piece of work. For a few, the actual touching of the work, imbued with meaning, can be experienced as a form of release. One can also be sensitized to a heightened degree of preciousness in the art work. Breaking this spell also permits the patient to boldly strike out in new directions and not be a party to his own internal

narcissistic restrictions. However, when the narcissistic investment is
in the work of art, the patient may be psychically wounded or de-
bilitated if the therapist physically touches it. A patient's perfectionism may well force him to come to a self-destructive position. The
work becomes his prison where he feels cut off and unrelated to
his inner self. A therapist may well protect the patient from this
position by helping him to walk away from his work in order to
approach it on another occasion with fresh eyes. Again, it is the art
therapist who must be in tune with the real rhythm of the energy so
he can combat the self-destructive introjects mobilized in the patient.

Thus, the alliance with the good mother is made, as the patient
fights off fears of retaliation that, at times, are manifested through
excessive perfectionism. The good mother in the art therapist encourages and protects, but also knows when to let go so that the
person can capture his own sense of power. The development of
autonomy is not only of importance between the patient and the
creative product but also between the patient and the therapist. A
therapist in tune with his patient will discern the process of individualization. As a person develops, he will need less and less psychic
nourishment until ultimately he is ready to explore new and different
environments. Separation can be very painful for both parties. The
beautiful sweetness, the intimacy, the power must be relinquished.
The patient makes a more realistic assessment of the therapist's
strengths and weaknesses. Possibly, both patient and therapist will
want to continue a contract that no longer services their individual
growth needs. Recognition of these feelings by the therapist demands
a good deal of depth and maturity. The patient in this developmental
stage will become angry at himself for his own unwillingness to
acknowledge separateness. Unless protected from himself, he may
become caught up in another introjective battle that can only con-
taminate, if not destroy, his work. In this instance, one sees literally
a wrenching apart that may be the ultimate requirement for gaining
freedom.

An art therapist has a highly sophisticated understanding of introjective processes (6). As was mentioned earlier in this chapter,
enormous untapped energies are bound up with introjects that are
stored deep within the recesses of the unconscious. As these introjects
emerge either within the relationship or in the artistic product, there
usually is a release of enormous energy that functions as an inspiration
for the creative act. These introjects can be experienced by the

therapist as literally possessing him in the form of demons. The induced feelings associated with these introjects can encompass such affects as rage, despair, hopelessness, etc. These emotions, which are originally part of a parental or child self, must be integrated and understood by the therapist in order to maintain the continual flow and release of energies. To act out these externalized introjects could well cause a re-introjection and a recreation of the original trauma. The art therapist must maintain the strength of his own identity and still foster a primitive union, especially when he is working with people who have extreme pathology.

The therapist combats these introjects in himself and acts as a model for the patient to face some of his own primitive terror. As these conflicts originate in an early stage of development, a nonverbal, feeling experience is implied in the curative act rather than an intellectual or verbal response. Nevertheless, a theoretical conceptualization of this complex process contributes significantly to a resolution within the art therapist. Many of these notions have been intuitively incorporated by experienced art teachers and therapists. (A theoretical understanding may prove helpful to the art therapist who finds himself on a plateau with a patient.) Creativity is an area that requires breadth and depth of psychological perspective. Many of these analytic concepts cannot be fully assimilated unless personal emotional growth accompanies a cognitive education.

Today our society appears to have produced increasing numbers of technicians with a high degree of information and competence. Of equal importance, however, is the development of talent that can deal creatively with complex problems that are part of a very complex society. Research seems to indicate that with more schooling and education, creativity in children is either cut off or destroyed. This may be a consequence of both the kind of teachers we have as well as the institutions that demand conformity and a particular kind of adjustment on the part of both teacher and pupil. Thus, the area that may ultimately prove most challenging, if not most fruitful, for art therapy may be in normal settings such as schools and settlement houses where children and adults can rediscover a lost part of themselves (7). In the interim, the art therapist will continue to make a valuable contribution to creativity development in hospitals and other mental health care settings. The depth and strength of his work in this area will be determined by a sophisticated knowledge of nonverbal communication, intrapsychic processes, and ego development.

References

1. Kris, E. *Psychoanalytic Explorations in Art*. New York: International Universities Press, 1952.
2. This point of view has been amplified in an unpublished paper presented by Dr. Alan Roland at the 1st Theodor Reik Center Conference, May, 1969, New York.
3. Spitz, R. A. *The First Year of Life*. New York: International Universities Press, 1965.
4. Noyd, P. "The Development of Music Ability." *The Psychoanalytic Study of the Child*. 23: 332–347, 1968.
5. Barron, F. "The Dream of Art and Poetry." *Psychology Today*. Vol. 2, No. 7, 18–29, 1968.
6. Bychowski, G. "Struggle Against the Introjects." *International Journal of Psychoanalysis*. Vol. 39, 327–330, 1958.
7. Haimowitz, H. *Human Development*. New York: Crowell, 1960. pp. 44–55.

5. Imagery: Part I

Picture if you will a group of art therapy students sitting in a small seminar. They are meeting in my living room. The room is small and we are aware of one another in spite of ourselves. Some are sitting on chairs, others are sitting on the floor. At first there is a tense expectant air in the room. No one speaks. I look, I wait and wonder what is going to happen. I feel somewhat tense myself. I feel myself to be pushy and controlling. The students in the group have been aware of this, and have reacted in the past in kind. Now this imago of my past, this dominating, controlling figure, lies somewhat subdued as a stronger sense of me loosens up and springs towards freedom. This is our last session for the year and the reports are due. Then quietly and poignantly one of the students states that he has something to read. Slowly a volley of poetic images and perceptions flow forth as he describes his work with a young boy. I will include part of this report by Pierre Boenig. But first a few comments. Pierre works in a school for emotionally disturbed children and his report describes the inner life experience of his work with a particular child. I will not attempt to give any of the history but offer to you one paragraph of his report which so much describes what we have been working towards.

> Mark goes with me to get my coffee, pours the coffee and then spits in the cup. Exploring the hallway further and further, visiting the class across the hall for a few minutes, hiding when strangers come into our room or trying to kick them out, cursing anyone inside or outside, demanding to be carried. Now I am walking, protecting, stopping, holding, comforting, an ally; fighting, killing and being killed; and also I am the strength, the power where frustration, anger, fear cries and tears mix, and melt through my acceptance of him. How much is it me, how much is it him? I give my resources, he gives his will to fight

Reprinted, with revisions, with permission from *Art Psychotherapy: An International Journal*, Vol. 1, Number 3/4: Winter 1973. Pergamon Press, New York.

the suffocation, the rigidity, the conformity, and all of a sudden he is by himself, with himself, his face dry.

Two days ago I told Mark that his mother would be coming to visit. For two days he worries what she will do to his position in the school. Now I tell him that when she comes I will be on his side, by his side. When mother came into the room Mark was on my lap, on the floor. He, his face on me, and I held him. He cried and screamed at her to get out, to leave. She told him not to cry, to be a good boy and if he would stop crying she would leave. She threw him kisses and looked paler than I had remembered her. Mark hid in my lap, crying so he could not hear what she had to say, wanting her out, away, out of the confusion, the fusion.

After hearing the report, the students are moved and deeply touched. I am particularly pleased as it graphically summarizes the course. Sometimes all of us wondered whether we were participants in a group therapy seminar. This didactic, somewhat overbearing imago in me would often put a stop to the flow of material and once again place us more certainly in a classroom atmosphere. However nebulous our subject, whatever the anxieties and tensions that accrued between us, all of us realized that we had shared an experience.

As I reviewed the course, one thing seemed to stand out. Art was play and all of us started to relearn how to play (1). Our orientation was not on a conscious, goal-directed level. Indeed we sought and drifted to a different level of existence—a shift in ego state, if you will, where we were able to tolerate the paradoxes and ambiguities of our thoughts. We encountered demons of our past, images of lost days and nights that seemed to contain untapped reservoirs of energy. I would like to talk briefly about these demons or introjects and relate them to what goes on in the creative dialogue.

All of us at one time or another appear to be captured by an introject. Often they creep up on us and literally transpose us so that we lose ourselves completely. These figures are like foreign islands within the deep reaches of our unconscious and represent the figurative embodiment of our personal lost battles and traumas. They have their own independent existence with a whole set of concomitant values, perceptions and notions. These island figures are not integrated into a unified self but emerge from time to time and completely dominate our thinking and behavior, if only momentarily.

The prescription for growth often calls upon us to face crises.

Through various developmental conflicts and encounters, key individuals in our past who are associated with these crises are incorporated fully into ourselves, for this is the result of an inability to separate and experience loss. For others, the feeling of being overwhelmed by either hostile or sexual impulses is too much for the child's self to cope with. They submit to the larger force and become one with it, losing the true self while the quest for identity is crippled. For many, these introjects have damaged the entire ego and we experience in our relationship with them a conglomeration of disintegrated imagos that has no central force or direction. Fortunately, there exists a reparative need to challenge these past devils and demons by externalizing them on a welter of different relationships. Sadly enough, the uncanny power of these introjects pushes the individual to recreate not only the same conflict of his past but also the same result. Thus, for some, human relationships are all too dangerous and fantasy and unconscious processes become the focus of emotional investment. For a fortunate few, the world of creativity becomes a major source of externalization. Here in the safety and confines of a sphere where they are completely in charge, the individual dares to bring forth and concretize the early representations of past conflicts.

Perhaps if I start this description of a journey into the unconscious with the very disturbed and distraught, it will provide a frame of reference that can be easily transferred to a wide range of patients. As I approach this patient immersed in his own world where there has been damage in many areas of perception, affects and integration, I search for the right melody to tune in to. For some, I can be but an extension and impose little of my own self or existence. I stand on the outside and observe. As I lose some of my own conscious control, I constantly seek ways of blending into this totality. Gradually I discover the various nonverbal roots that can establish this very early form of relatedness. I attempt to pick up on the most sensitive level of the patient's primary sense of rhythm and touch. Indeed, I hope I may be to the patient as a sensitive mother who approaches a young child who has been brutalized.

In many respects I witness and feel the beginning of a love relationship. Yet, as the patient dares to explore on this primary journey that is mediated through graphic play, I observe that something strange is taking hold of me. Seemingly, from out of nowhere, the terror and hell of the patient's infant self are felt within me.

I experience the parental forces that existed in the patient's past.

The long-felt contempt, disdain or ambivalence possesses me like a demon. I now know, on a feeling level, what this patient has gone through in his early life. To have the courage not to act out this externalized introject with the patient, to be able to maintain my sense of self and at the same time allow myself to be engulfed by these feelings puts a tremendous burden on me. But, if I can show him that I will not be overwhelmed or lose myself to these devils, perhaps then the patient will learn from me and internalize my strength. Perhaps I, too, would try to harness this force through my own personal art work. I will have to decide whether the patient is ready and willing to see what I experience with him. Maybe all that is necessary is to feel deeply what is going on in the patient. This, in and of itself, is a communication. For where there is a deep sense of injury, part of the reparative work is to feel what the patient has felt in the past. Together we experience pain, rage, and a welter of affects. Involved in this curative as well as creative process, there is a release of energy. As one introject subsides, another looms up for both of us to encounter and experience. Over and over again I creatively attempt to assess the distance and closeness of our relationship and determine the dosage that the patient can take of what I have to offer. At the same time, I am very much aware of my own personal battles and demons and try to separate them from the art therapy relationship. What I do relate to has much more to do with what is induced by the patient and his work.

I encounter some difficulty in determining the kind and amount of images I choose to share with a patient. Some patients experience a sense of intrusion if there is any mutuality. In these instances, I wait until enough time has passed so he can test out his terrors within the more protective confines of his art work. I wait for an invitation. If none is forthcoming, I wonder if there are feelings inside of me that are interfering in our relationship. On the other hand, there are some who will only enter into an art therapy dialogue when and if I make the first overture. For a few, a self-portrait may be the invitation required of me so that the overture can begin. Others might be intrigued or touched by a graphic gift. Each has his own starting point and demands all the consideration and thought that goes on in good child-rearing.

In graphically expressing my own imagery, I am careful not to overwhelm the patient by my skill. Indeed, I show my past errors and ask for help. At the same time, it is important that I not be a phony, for he will sense this immediately.

I deal with art imagery in myself differently, depending on the particular problem or issue at hand. I think of the very deprived child. The child that has minimal identification and a vacuum inside of him speaks of an empty breast. Though he seems depressed, more accurately he is empty. My imagery and fantasies are used as a source of stimulation and engagement and at the same time supply the raw food for ego building. I can think of no better way of developing a sense of self than through sharing my imagery with the child. In contrast to the child who has been overwhelmed by a parent, this one will selectively take from me the images and fantasies that will enhance his own sense of genetic destiny.

A patient may make contact with himself and learn through a mirror reflection of his own psychic processes. The direct confrontation and verbal dialogue are experienced as wounding. I think in particular of persons with character disorders who fend off anything that is strange or foreign. In these instances, I may outdo the patient's imagery and exaggerate his defenses, while giving him distance and control.

One of the areas that lends itself very well to the use of mutual imagery sharing is work with children. Together we enter a world of fantasy and play. We exchange roles, models, and imagos. Together we loosen up, allow our fantasies to travel, and join in the art work. Sometimes I cannot do this. I must wait for consolidation of the ego that occurs through the art work before I can go on.

Yet play therapy should not be confined to children. Playing with fantasies and images is what art is all about. Adults may need a chance to act out, in the safe confines of a therapeutic relationship, where there is a joint living out of imagos and roles and there can be some release of inhibition and constraint.

As I view the art therapy relationship and its dialogue, the horizons that both patient and therapist can cross appear boundless. The limitation of this journey may well be the therapist's capacity to experience a whole range of difficult and complex feelings that may accrue either from the patient or from himself.

I view the art therapist of the future essentially as a specialist in the creative process. Images and symbols are the everyday language of creativity. The art therapist understands the power of the symbol and utilizes this tool as a very special way of communicating. He recognizes that the image pulls together many levels of the psyche and can make a more accurate and complex statement of cognition than any verbal interpretation.

References

1. Horowitz, M. J. *Image Formation and Cognition.* New York: Appleton-Century-Crofts, 1970.

6. Imagery: Part II

by Julie Joslyn Brown and
Arthur Robbins

Introduction

The purpose of this chapter is to present a theoretical and experiential view of the use of the art therapist's imagery in the therapeutic process. We contend that the use of imagery is a powerful tool which has been underutilized and not fully understood, and hope to demonstrate how the therapist's preconscious can be used for depth interpretations, resistance analysis and symbiotic relatedness. All too often, the therapist faces powerful primitive material that she cannot readily respond to verbally. Indeed, words are often insufficient for connection on the primitive level that is necessary for depth communication with chronic, regressed or psychotic patients. In addition, the use of the therapist's imagery as a response to the therapeutic process may well even have applicability to neurotic and characterological cases. This is particularly true when such patients are approaching pregenital issues.

In order to demonstrate this complex dialogue, we will attempt to give some sense of a therapeutic interaction through both metaphorical and visual imagery. Where appropriate the art work of the patient and of the therapist's response will be illustrated. You will also experience a verbal interchange representing the *preconscious* experience of both participants. However, it is important to emphasize that even the poetic image cannot duplicate what occurs on a preverbal level with such patients. After each particular example of a visual and metaphorical exchange, the authors will then attempt to clarify some of the underlying dynamics between therapist and patient.

Case 1: Sam

The first case deals with a 55-year-old man who has been hospitalized for the better part of 30 to 35 years. He presents a chronic psychotic picture characterized by incontinence, withdrawal, obsessive rumination and a primitive, archaic style of thinking. At this particular point in treatment, Sam, after showing some signs of growth and contact, panicked with marked decompensation of defenses. His incontinence on the ward was more frequent and his art productions more primitive. He began resisting and withholding; he was angry and often sadistic. His degree of fragmentation and restlessness intensified. In the following exchanges, which, we should emphasize, represent communication on a preconscious level, you will see examples of unsuccessful, as well as more appropriate, use of imagery as a therapeutic response to the patient.

Interchange 1

> PATIENT: I'm falling, I'm biting, I'm shitting; drowning—helping—lost—confusion. Shit. Where are you? I feel full, empty, lost, I need. I don't know. Where are you?
> THERAPIST: I'm here. Here I am. Look at me!
> PATIENT: Shit.
> THERAPIST: Look at me.
> PATIENT: Piss.
> THERAPIST: Look at me. I'm human. Me. Look.
> PATIENT: Lost. I know nothing. I'm hungry. Give me something.
> THERAPIST: I'm here—living, breathing, loving. Let me love you.
> PATIENT: Crap. Everything gone, debris. I eat. Go away—
> THERAPIST: Everything gone, everything lost.
> PATIENT: Everything lost. Go away. Play.
> THERAPIST: I'm falling. I'm falling.
> PATIENT: I'm playing, shit. Swim.

Together

> THERAPIST: I'm swimming and shitting.
> PATIENT: Crapping.
> THERAPIST: Shitting.
> PATIENT: Crapping. Playing. I'm lost.
> THERAPIST: I'm helpless.
> PATIENT: I'm hungry.

THERAPIST: Falling.
PATIENT: Nowhere.
PATIENT: Nowhere. . . . I am here.
THERAPIST: I am here.

In this example, Sam was lost in a morass of undifferentiated thoughts and feelings and yet woefully disconnected from his own feelings and the world around him. The therapist, in an attempt to gain contact with the patient in his mass of confusion, presents herself as human, demanding recognition and response on a mature adult level. She presents him with a gift of a clay human head (Figure 6.1, see Color Illustration, p. A), proclaiming her availability, which could not possibly be received by the patient, who was at this point deep into his regression (Figure 6.2, see Color Illustration, p. A). When the therapist was able to relate on an equally primitive level, contact became possible. The therapist's second gift (Figure 6.3, see Color Illustration, p. A), an unformed mass of clay, even smaller and less defined than Sam's clay form, served to connect the two. It should be noted that the therapist's response was neither contrived nor preconceived. The image evolved out of her own preconscious relatedness to the patient's emotional state, reflecting her frustration and despair.

Thus, the therapist was able to allow her own primary thought process to break through and join the patient via her own art work. Her mass of clay symbolized the diffusion of impulses and feelings as well as the fragmentation that the patient was undergoing. This, we believe, is an important step for such a regressed patient towards ego reconstruction and the development of any sense of self and individuality.

The next interchange reflects another phase of treatment. Here Sam was less involved in an infantile regression, developing some sense of separateness from the therapist and increasing his ability to feel tenderness. Of further note, the patient's motor involvement with clay progressed from a characteristically infantile bilaterally symmetrical pinching motion to a more complicated set of hand movements.

Interchange 2

PATIENT: It feels. It feels like sand, it feels wet. But look, something smooth and round. Look what I've done. It almost feels alive. I remember something long ago. I almost hear something. Oh? I almost hear, long ago, something lost.

Something round, something smooth. I can touch.

THERAPIST: Yes, something smooth. Something slippery.

PATIENT: I almost know. I can almost hear you, but I won't look.

THERAPIST: Keep safe. Keep warm. Keep smooth. I am here and I am quiet.

PATIENT: Dare I touch? Dare I feel? It almost feels like I'm alive.

Part of the process of reintegration in a chronic psychotic patient involves rediscovering the senses, specifically the sense of tenderness, present in the early relatedness of mother and child. The therapist's clay image—a solid and smooth mound—attempts to communicate a sense of quiet, security and protection. Thus patient and therapist resonate the beginnings of a relationship that has some elements of trust and care providing the raw fuel for future growth and discovery.

The next group of photographs demonstrates the therapist's use of herself as a provocative agent. She has had enough of Sam's regression. Here we see illustrated through imagery and metaphor a confrontation and challenge for a more frontal expression of the patient's sadism.

Interchange 3

THERAPIST: Here I am, I'm a woman. I have big breasts: I'm different from you.

PATIENT: I'll tear and rip. I hate those fucking breasts. I'll rip and show. I'll show the world where it's really at. I'll show the bullet and I'll show the gun. I hate that fuckin' woman's breasts.

THERAPIST: I'm still a woman.

PATIENT: You put on the arms.

THERAPIST: Here are my arms to hold you.

PATIENT: I'll put on the head. But I'll make myself in my own image ... You goddamn woman. You won't take me with those breasts.

THERAPIST: But I'm still a woman.

PATIENT: And I've got a penis. So leave my penis and I'll leave your breasts. Don't you dare take—

In this example, the therapist presents a strongly individuated image of her self and offers this symbol to the patient (Figure 6.4, see Color

Illustration, p. B). The patient at first sees only a part of the totality that is the therapist. At this point he threatens to rip off the breasts of the clay figure. Only through the releasing of destructive energies towards the symbol representing his frustration, the breast, was he able to start separating himself out from an undifferentiated mass. As they jointly create the figure the patient adds male genitals. Thus, the therapist provides a vehicle for the release of primitive sadistic impulses, resulting in reconstruction and increased self-definition, assertion of sexual identity and greater integration. Within this self-affirmation, he tenuously rediscovers a male part of himself, but still defends against his own projected cannibalistic impulses.

The next interchange demonstrates the therapist's decision to work in a more goal-directed, structured, and reality-oriented manner. The therapist gives very specific instructions as to the modeling of the clay dog.

Interchange 4

> THERAPIST: Now make the legs. Make one leg at a time. First the front legs . . .
> PATIENT: God she's showing me where the legs are. There's walls, some order, I got something to hold on to.
> THERAPIST: Now make the back legs, touch them. Touch them.
> PATIENT: There's the back. There's the front.
> THERAPIST: Make the legs stronger. One leg at a time. I feel my own legs lengthen.
> PATIENT: I almost feel the leg. I almost feel. She's showing me where I am. I can almost feel that I have legs: that I have arms. Thank God she's around. I feel almost held.

In this particular phase of treatment, an unstructured symbiotic form of relatedness is no longer needed. Sam begins to respond to the reality proddings of the therapist. She insists upon a realistic and functional replication of a dog. The patient feels relieved to have some structure to function within. At an earlier point of treatment this approach would have made little impact, since the symbiotic interchange was necessary as a foundation for growth.

The therapist structures reality and thus helps the patient discover the self through exploration of the body image, via the sculpture of the dog. As a mother would reflect and mirror back, as well as contain and structure, the child, the therapist helps Sam begin to gain a sense of his body as an integrated and functioning totality, that is likewise connected to the world around him. We see in this particular instance secondary process skills utilized by the therapist within a primary relatedness.

Case 2: Davey

The next case concerns a 28-year-old hospitalized man in a state of diffuse panic. He presented a disconnected, infantile and bizarre picture to the entire staff. At this particular juncture in the therapeutic relationship, erotic and sadistic impulses were breaking through to the preconscious level, causing panic and increased regression, evident in the art work. Again, the following interchange represents intense feelings which have been translated into words here to clarify the imagery.

Interchange 5

> PATIENT: Penis, scumbag, cut . . . rip. I don't know. Pictures, walls, therapist cut. Stupid. Get me out of here. Cut. I've got a penis . . . What's going on? Get me out. Walls, tables, chairs. Penis. Schmuck. You want to play little girl? You want to see my pee pee. Shit on you. Play with it—work it over. Too bad. Walls. Sticks. You want to play? I'd bet you'd be interested. Walls. Pee pee. Ha Ha! Where's everybody?
>
> THERAPIST: (shouting) Help. Get me out of this fucking place. I'm growing up. I can't stand it anymore. Let me be born. Help me. Cut me loose. I'm suffocating.

This is an excellent example of how the art therapist's art work can break through countertransference defenses. In the sessions, the patient was hostile, sadistic, acting out on an infantile level, and yet cut off from his own feelings. He was too agitated to participate in any creative process. The therapist was out of touch with the patient's underlying panic. However, through the drawings, at a subsequent point, she was able to understand the full force of his feelings.

In this particular presentation, we see too levels of relatedness within the therapist. On the more conscious level she felt extreme frustration with and isolation from the patient. Yet, on a deeper level, her art imagery (Figure 6.5, see Color Illustration, p. B) connects with the real unconscious communication of the patient—his sense of panic and intolerable fear. In the actual session the therapist felt shut out and disconnected. Undoubtedly the affects were so powerful that she was unable to connect with the utter rawness of his distress. Later, like fragments of a dream, her drawings of the session connect her with the real impact of the therapeutic encounter.

Case 3: Josephine

The following case presents a 28-year-old chronic psychotic woman who, upon entering the hospital, was in a state of extreme catatonic excitement. She was explosive, vitriolic, violent and assaultive. Now, after months of treatment, primitive material of a largely symbiotic nature is being reworked and reintegrated. On occasion, as in the first group of illustrations, the therapist faces a good deal of denial.

Interchange 6

> PATIENT: Clip-top. Everything tight.
>   boxes, squares—everything right.
>   Boxes, squares, hearts in the middle—
>   Everything is square. Everything is right.
> THERAPIST: I'm bleeding. I'm bleeding.
>   Where is this coming from?
>   Where is this blood coming from?
>   I feel like I'm being nailed to a cross. Holes in hands, throat cut.
> PATIENT: Clip-top. Everything's right.
> THERAPIST: Everything's *not* right.
>   I'm bleeding!
> PATIENT: Isn't that right? Wouldn't you right. Rather be tight. Wouldn't I like to see your face full of blood?

In this particular instance the therapist somewhere felt the patient's underlying hostility. Only through the therapist's art production was the unconscious interchange clarified. The patient offers the therapist a guarded and defensive drawing (Figure 6.6, see Color Illustration, p. B). The therapist's imagery, with its blood-red jagged lines (Figure 6.7, see Color Illustration, p. C), is shared subsequently with the patient. In fact, the therapist was not at all in touch with what the patient produced in her. Only after the spontaneous production of the art imagery could she contact these deep feelings. Again, this imagery was neither contrived nor conscious. Though the therapist often takes a supportive and non-intrusive stance, here she unconsciously subverts the defense and responds to the id material. As a consequence, without any verbal interpretations from the therapist, the patient becomes more connected on a conscious level to her sadism.

The visual imagery of the therapist is utilized on a very preconscious level: She allows something to happen within her, and thus, after the fact, discovers via the patient's own interpretation the meaning of her response. Interestingly, the communication originated on an unconscious level in the patient, became preconscious in the therapist, and through imagery of the therapist, the patient was finally able to make her own interpretation by saying: "I came down to torture you."

The next illustration reflects an interaction between therapist and patient in the same art work. It takes place as the patient undergoes a volley of manic defenses. She grabs the art therapist's work and scribbles an addition.

Interchange 7

    PATIENT: Come on in boys! Come on in girls!
        Let's fill up this room. Sit here, sit there. Get on my lap. How are you kitchy poo? Go fuck yourself, Julie. Come on in. Slam the door. Open your head. Everybody sit on Julie's fat ass.
    THERAPIST: I'll sit . . . and I'll be waiting.

In some phases, while working with regressed psychotics, the problems of distance and closeness ebb and flow with each level of integration. Thus, the therapist must be constantly alerted to fears of closeness and must be able to give the appropriate therapeutic response. In Josephine's case, closeness means merging and loss of self. Through the drawings and visual interplay, the therapist breaks through her distancing techniques and calmly offers herself as an object for intimacy without trying to overwhelm the patient's fragile ego resources. At this time, the patient utilizes manic defenses and the therapist offers a womb-like enveloping image. The patient listens and responds verbally, lets closeness happen and gives up her defensive posture. She is finally able to arrive at her own interpretation for the newly forming symbiotic relatedness: "What's that? An ocean and an amoeba? Osmosis . . . osmosis." In this particular symbolic interplay, patient and therapist relate through the same drawing (Figure 6.8, see Color Illustration, p. C) where clearly Josephine encases her therapist and strengthens the cord between them. This is accomplished symbolically and visually by Josephine's reinforcing the connection between the "amoeba" and the "ocean." She also adds a black blazing sun, a reminder of the terror of overwhelming intimacy.

In the next example you will see an inappropriate violation of the patient's autonomous needs when the therapist imposes her imagery on the patient. Here the patient accepts the image as a valid response to her conflict regarding closeness, symbiotic relatedness and fears of self-destruction. Again, in the following example, the picture (Figure 6.9, see Color Illustration, p. C) is a joint one between ait therapist and patient.

Interchange 8

> THERAPIST: I see a wall between us. I can't touch you. I can't feel you. I feel terribly disconnected. Blocked, stopped, afraid.
>
> PATIENT: I'm on my way. Get out of my way. I know you're here. You've been good, but I'm on my way.
>
> THERAPIST: Where are you?
>
> PATIENT: Don't you understand? Please don't hold me. Let me go. I love you. I care for you. But let me go.
>
> THERAPIST: It's hard to let go.
>
> PATIENT: You can do it. Let me go. I'm on my way. Stay over here.

In this instance the therapist responds to her own needs for contact in connection with the patient's need for individuation. The imagery and associations of the therapist are functions of her own needs rather than a response to the symbolic communication of the patient. At first the therapist attempts to demonstrate to the patient how cut off she feels by seeing her parallel lines only as a wall severing the connection between them. In the course of the session, the therapist becomes more in tune with the patient and experiences her parallel lines now as "railroad tracks" leading her to a journey toward self-definition and independence.

The therapist illustrates one of the values of the use of her own visual imagery. She has a chance to study and reexperience the symbolic interplay over a period of time to discover the appropriate level of patient-therapist relatedness.

Imagery in a Group Dialogue

Up to this point we have given illustrations of individual patient-therapist encounters. Our last example will hopefully demonstrate how the therapist uses herself in a group situation. The following group met several times previously and at this point in its development conspired to conceal and deny the anger and explosiveness lying dormant in the mural (Figure 6.10, see Color Illustration, p. D). At first the members of the group completely ignored the explosive hostile symbols within the group. No one paid any attention to the bombs and planes. Some members in fact tried to conceal the bombs behind clouds. The therapist decided that somewhere, somehow, the explosiveness and anger had to be accepted or at least integrated within the total group pattern. She decided that she had to be the unspoken voice within the group, the one with the courage to come and confront what others needed to deny. The therapist let the bomb fall, drawing in an explosion. The group was then forced into confronting the anger and hostility and embarked on either rescue efforts or participation in the destruction, exploring the group's true feelings. With the therapist as facilitator, the group was able to progress from a fairly superficial, disintegrated, defensive position, to a more threatening one, but also a more accurate and real one.

Conclusion

The authors have attempted to give but a few examples of the use of their own imagery as a means of making therapeutic contact with highly regressed patients. Imagery can be used as a form of symbiotic relatedness, as a way of breaking through defenses, and as an interpretive form of contact so that patients can become more connected to disconnected parts of themselves.

As a therapist explores the deeper reaches of patient's relatedness and dissociation, the verbal interchange seems woefully inadequate to make contact with such primitive, archaic forces. Patients at this level need to feel, touch and see, if not visually experience, themselves through the therapist's relationship. The art therapist has a very special and valid tool that she can apply within the therapeutic scene. It would seem to us the use of symbolic play strikes near the essence of what an art therapist offers at the most complex and richest levels of communication.

There are obviously many cautions which need to be stated in the use of this approach to patients. Primary process material does not always lead to a greater understanding of the self. Often this material avoids any real quest for connection and serves resistance. A therapist must be intensely aware of some of the unconscious forces within her. If nothing else, she must have the courage to look at the very essence of what she is all about. These patients will undoubtedly touch and play with the most primitive reaches of the therapist's unconscious sense of herself. A therapist who is unable or too threatened to approach this level is wiser to use art as a means of sublimation, restricting herself to dealing with secondary process material.

The authors cannot overemphasize the potential danger inherent in sharing one's personal imagery with a patient. It is not a technique to be used indiscriminately. The beginning student who may not feel at home with his own unconscious processes may tend to utilize this technique as a means to undermine, rather than facilitate, the treatment. Close supervision becomes a necessity.

We would also stress that symbiotic relatedness does not mean that the therapist fuses with his patient. A delicate interchange occurs wherein the therapist preserves his autonomy and yet is able to identify and empathize completely with the patient. Because this process requires an access to primitive areas within the therapist's psyche, there is a potential danger for the therapist to lose his own ego boundaries. This loss of control is both contraindicated and antitherapeutic.

We believe there exists room for more dynamic use of art within the therapeutic relationship. We see the creative part of art therapy as one in which imagery flows between patient and therapist, where art materials function as a bridge—a bridge where symbolism reaches out and enhances a therapeutic process. Art materials are used in a very dynamic sense. The materials only provide a means for expressing symbolism—symbolism that can lead the process further into self-discovery. Basically, we are referring to "process"—a fluid and ongoing process where the imagery of the therapist connects, stimulates, responds to, mirrors and interprets an increasing sense of self-realization. We do not see art therapy stagnating the process through "polished" concrete productions or through stock questions and answers of a diagnostic origin. All too often art therapists are warned to stay away from primary process material. They are told to build the ego and strengthen the patient's sense of reality. Ego-building, however, would seem to occur when the self becomes more connected to its various disconnected parts. We have here attempted to present a therapeutic approach which integrates fragmented part-images into a more complete whole. We contend that the art therapist must have a thorough and profound sense of dynamics, as well as a sensitive understanding of therapeutic process, a familiarity with imagery, and the openness and skill to harness material in a meaningful exchange.

7. Clinical Considerations

To an entering student, imbued with the beauty of artistic expression and fantasy play, there is nothing more important than offering patients creative experiences to unleash them from personal emotional prisons. Slowly, however, this goal is perceived as inadequate and naive. When some patients do not grow, and others misuse or abuse therapeutic overtures, something more is needed. A belief in nonverbal communication is simply not enough—a hard look into the specific therapeutic issues presented by various patient groups is in order.

This chapter cannot substitute for intensive readings in personality dynamics and treatment techniques. As a student masters these readings, she may apply her tools to facilitate creative movement and change. However, the foregoing material assumes that the student has a clinical framework. We hope here to provide a broad synthesis of treatment technique as applied specifically to nonverbal expression.

As a beginning, we must consider the emotional currents that affect our treatment stance. Can you visualize a patient's ego, with its capacity to handle pressures from within and without? Is it rigid, like a tightly bound fortress? Could it crumble like a sand castle if you apply extra pressure? What is the nature or character of the defenses that surround the self? Perhaps denial or repression; or a fluid mixture of adaptive devices in and out. Maybe a drawing or another visualization of this experience is appropriate. Can you imagine a figurative representation of your patient's character style? A myriad of images may arise that gives an essence of the patient, as well as a conception to construct a self, an ego, and a network of defenses.

There is much more to assess and weigh. Can you feel yourself emerge in the pattern of transference communications? Does the patient let you exist as a separate entity or does he distort and mold you into an extension of his narcissistic self? What about the real relationship? Are you a builder . . . a shield . . . or perhaps a mediator for a fractured ego? Does the patient allow you to lend part of your strengths and resources to cope with the world? Is the patient drowning but refusing your lifeline as he starts to go down again?

Each broad grouping of patient behavior presents characteristic issues for the art therapist. The following diagnostic positions can be helpful in formulating a treatment plan. However, we cannot emphasize enough that the following descriptions are merely guidelines. No one patient ever falls clearly into any one diagnostic category. Each person is a unique entity with a multitude of characterological styles and must be seen as "original," as through the eyes of an artist. These guidelines are not intended to restrict the vision of the student but to help her more easily understand the singular reality of each individual patient.

Clinical references that offer more complete discussions of individual diagnostic groupings appear at the end of this chapter.

Neurological Disorders ✓

The broad spectrum of neurological disabilities offers a good starting point. The patient with a neurological disorder tends to be hyperactive, excitable, emotionally labile, and distractable; his thinking processes tend toward concretism. He presents such perceptual difficulties as perseveration and a diminished capacity to distinguish figure from ground. This characterization has certain implications for an educational-therapeutic point of view and approach. Presented material should be concrete, structured and defined. Stimulation should be minimized and psychomotor coordination demands kept fairly simple. While bright, alive and multivariegated colors are at first avoided, poster paints rather than oils or finger paints seem more suitable. Clay, if introduced, should be presented in small amounts. The therapist provides patients with instructions from the rudimentary gradually to the more complex.

Educational and rehabilitative approaches often stop at this juncture, with the entire emphasis on perceptual training and organization (2). By implication, all that is needed is retraining. Self-exploration, fantasy play, and creative expression are often seen as interferences to this learning process. Yet, this myopic view deceives. On closer inspection this patient is confused as to his body image and has all the attending developmental living problems. If anything, his emotional life is further complicated by perceptual difficulties that cannot be solved simply by conditioning, structure, and retraining. The art therapist, cognizant of the perceptual needs and limitations of his patients, gradually enlarges the neurologically handicapped person's capacity to handle expressive communication. Dosage and timing go hand in hand with a slow building of release techniques.

Try to picture yourself as an art therapist with a group of brain-damaged children. The room is booming and buzzing like a beehive, crackling with impulses and energy.

Clearly functioning as a role model, you gradually introduce simple, structured activities that capture this energy. Later, working with an individual child, you might offer more expressive art materials for the child to explore and investigate. You build, increase and reinforce frustration tolerance. Within the security of a safe and clear world, the child takes a chance and begins to confront some of his inner life material. He experiences the joy of mastery as well as the thrill of creation. Imagination and fantasy are no longer bottled up or over-looked but given an outlet through the art work.

Once the mode for creative expression has been established there are many areas to explore. The body image is investigated through tracing techniques and clay work, while perceptual diffusion and feelings of social inadequacy and impotency are brought forth through a host of play techniques. Feelings of perplexity and impotence may be conceptualized through nonverbal media. In more serious neuro-logical cases, the patient may not have the verbal tools to describe the sense of chaos and confusion. The clear and concrete representa-tions of feeling states may be one way of making this situation some-what easier to handle (1, 2).

Mental Retardation

Art therapy makes a unique contribution to mentally retarded chil-dren and adults. The world of fantasy and creative play is a vista not often crossed by these patients when placed in the ordinary institu-tional settings. Mental retardation does not necessarily imply an equal retardation in the capacity for creative and imaginative work. Yet, retarded patients may be shunted into back wards with minimal stimulation and communication. Art therapy offers an opportunity to open up a whole new life of images, sensations and feelings, potentially making the difference between stagnation and vitality.

With the mentally retarded patient the practitioner starts on the sensory level in order to acquaint patients with feelings and sensations that establish the pattern for an inner life. Expression should not be restricted to one sense modality. Music, dance, and drama, along with art, are necessary ingredients to lay the groundwork for translations into imaginative experiences.

This patient literally hungers for attention and care. Once the art therapist gives this attention, her creativity is constantly challenged to explore the appropriate sensory level that moves this patient into imaginative spaces. The therapist introduces each activity slowly so that the experience becomes familiar and concrete. For instance, touching of the various parts of the body of one another as well as the therapist can be constantly repeated before progressing to body tracing exercises. Concurrently, one might also use mirrors, polaroid cameras or videotape to enhance the visual feedback. Music or dance helps facilitate the assimilation process by furthering the exploration of the rhythm and movement of one's body.

A wide range of encounter touch techniques are integrated with educational, ego-building and reinforcement theory. Lack of stimulation certainly may regress the intellectual functioning of mentally retarded patients. This group deserves the opportunity not only to feel and be touched but also to learn how to play and feel alive (3).

Geriatrics

Working with the elderly can be a meaningful experience for the art therapist. Expressionless faces on immobile bodies cry, "Listen and respect me; value what I have to offer. Do not discard me for there is worth in what I have to contribute." Often this message is not heard or responded to. The older person can be found sitting alone, having minimal interaction with his world. Institutions reinforce this dysphoric experience, by caring for patients with marginal enthusiasm and even less understanding of their needs.

At the very least, an art therapist can be open and available for an involved and feeling relationship. In many instances, the elderly need much more. A strong developmental need may exist to put life in order, to reflect and to make a statement about the individual life experience. Art therapy may offer an opportunity for a pictorial overview, capturing feelings of loss, separation and disconnection as well as those of joy, love and accomplishment. Images and traces long since without words float together through the art experience. At times, the visualization of a life cycle produces a good deal of discussion and introspection. But for many, the picture may say it all, requiring no explication.

The elderly person may find it difficult to deal with abstractions or material without something concrete and familiar to hold onto. At first he may need to relate on an arts and crafts level so his products become gifts that function as a connection to friends and relatives. These products ultimately may be a transition point for more imaginative work. Another patient, however, may need to maintain ties to his neighborhood or community. In these instances, the art therapist moves past the limitations imposed by an art room and evolves into a creative social facilitator. For example, children and young adults need the wisdom and love of the elderly; likewise, some older adults need to share the joy and exuberance of the young. The art therapist finds ways to set up activities such as exhibits, fairs and workshops. When the therapist creates a meeting ground for elders to find respect and meaning within the total community, the end of life becomes more of a fluid extension of a changing identity. Old age does not necessarily mean the end of growing. The creative sphere, characterized by a timeless quality, may give new meaning to those faced with death and separation. The imaginative and creative world can at least help make the transition to a state of cosmic unity (4).

Schizophrenia

The world of Picasso's *Guernica* is upon you as you encounter the reality of schizophrenia. Ravaged and pained forms, distorted phantoms and ghosts, confusion and panic float in and obscure your vision. The art therapist's very being is rocked as the power of unconscious symbols of the patient's faraway past are reactivated. The gloom and ache of lost battles and the piercing deadness of something empty and gone become present. Schizophrenia takes on many shapes and forms. However, all schizophrenics have in common a sense of defeat and retreat from external reality. For some, this loss virtually began at birth so that not even a glimmer of a self to be rediscovered or reborn is provided. There are chronic and acute patients, nondifferentiated patients, as well as more encapsulated patients with crystallized versions of pain and terror; their diagnoses read catatonic, paranoid, and hebephrenic. Each patient hopefully has a distillation of a self to be rediscovered, an ego to be regenerated, and a reality that needs reintroduction. The self within awaits contact. Perhaps art may be a way to find courage and hope by putting the various pieces of a fragmented self into a new whole.

In working with this group of patients, words often take on peculiar meanings. At times, they are experienced as an intrusion or an assault; they give little room to breathe. The picture or the nonverbal act gives a more open and less threatening space to explore. Life problems are on a preverbal level where the very textural quality of the art work promotes and encourages a form of symbiotic relatedness. Of primary importance is the art therapist's capacity to capture the rhythm and tempo of her patients. Art materials enhance the relationship, stimulating the externalization of introjects crucial in bringing about a reintegration. Slowly, the art therapist can tune into the pace and quality of the patient's life process. By engaging the unconscious and converting vague fears and affects into distinct images and pictures, the therapist and patient build an ego to harness, mediate and synthesize these energies into something comprehensible and communicable. The therapist lends her resources to make this journey less frightening for the patient, being careful to avoid stimulating a regression to fusion and nothingness.

Today an increasing number of hospital programs address themselves to the adaptive resources of the patient. The well-trained therapist combines resocialization techniques with her knowledge of unconscious symbolism and creates a flow in her work going from the unconscious to the conscious self, constantly encouraging an emerging identity. Thus the art therapist aids in organizing and synthesizing imagos and introjects and reinforces the emerging capacity of the patient to mold this material into a creative statement about himself.

Art therapists can also understand how and when expressive materials are used as a massive defense instead of a release for regeneration. Not all delusional or hallucinatory material is connected with the self. Much, in fact, protects and hides the self from emergence. The art therapist needs to understand when fantasy is a connection rather than a separation from the self. The art therapist's feelings provide a most important guide in making this distinction. Indeed, her feelings may be the only criterion that has any validity. Is she bored? Is she disconnected? Does the material feel stereotyped and flat? Or does she feel engaged and related to affects that either the material or the relationship induce? Thus, the art therapist can creatively use herself and materials with a very sophisticated understanding of ego and unconscious dynamics.

In many institutional settings, the art therapist may find herself increasingly preoccupied with the development of the ego functions of her patients. Art then becomes a safe testing ground where the patient tries out various alternative solutions for problem situations that are illuminated by the art experience. The ego functions of time, space and judgment, to name but a few, are closely scrutinized. This approach is particularly useful with chronic and pre-symbiotic patients who need constant building, reinforcing, and channeling of an adaptive ego.

An example of the above process is the execution of a clay model. The therapist helps the patient conceptualize and plan his work. She gives him an opportunity to verbalize his ideas as well as lay out step by step the means of carrying his plan into action. The model is constantly molded and remolded till the inner representation and the outer embodiment have some real meaning and communicative value. The therapist constantly reinforces the execution of the art work so that it makes sense not only to the patient but to others. At some point the schizophrenic must be able not only to depict his symbols and affects in the art work but somewhere find a road that makes contact with others rather than being a path to autistic withdrawal (5).

Psychosis

Psychotic patients may well be affected with disorders of the central nervous system. Various addictions can precipitate a break that has all the trappings of a functional disorder. However, when the etiological factors are brought to light, the central nervous system disorder becomes a paramount factor. Again, the many elements that relate to brain damage require the attention of the art therapist—structure, concretization and a carefully paced building of ego functions are needed.

Another common psychotic state can be found with patients suffering with manic-depressive psychosis. In these cases, the therapist avoids allowing patients to consume art materials voraciously. She attends the underlying depression and communicates through the art and through a close, supportive relationship. Art materials are consciously used to reach an underlying fear of loss and sense of blackness (6).

Neurosis

The neurotic is often all too aware of the world around him and handles it with at least a modicum of adaption. His defenses, to some degree, work for him. This sometimes comes at the cost of self-expression and an inner vitality. An art therapist brings a range of expressive techniques that are directed at emotional release. With neurotic patients therapy emphasizes emotional reaction, fantasy and play, focusing on the ability to respond. Feelings should not only be expressed but worked through so that there is a connection between the cognitive and emotional worlds.

An excellent contrast can be made between the obsessive and hysterical style of neurotic adaptation. The former is characterized by an isolation of affect, a predilection for power and control, and a belief in the magic of words and rationalizations. Art is an excellent vehicle to break through these intellectual controls. Think of the fastidious patient who is confronted with the dirt and mess of clay or the gushiness of finger paints, or perhaps the entanglement of armature wire. He cannot hide behind the word. The material demands a response. The work focuses upon synthesizing thinking and feeling functions. By contrast, patients with an hysterical emphasis rely on action and dramatization. There is emotional lability and an intolerance for anxiety; repression seems to be a major defense. The therapist helps patients connect words with affects. The approach then recognizes the cognitive problems of these patients by utilizing art as a stimulus for associations and insights.

With all neurotic patients, the art therapist needs to assess the character style that protects the intrapsychic conflict. Equally important, the cooperative aspects of the treatment relationship must be utilized. By the very nature of neurosis, as contrasted to psychosis, a cooperative ego exists. The therapist forms an alliance with the healthy part of the patient and works towards wholeness. Verbal and non-verbal modalities work in greater harmony. At times, there may be more talk than play. In other instances, art may break through resistances where more orthodox techniques have failed. The art therapist need not feel out of her element if the patient only wants to talk. Art experiences do not need to be contrived or forced; a creative experience can come through words as well as acts (7, 8).

Depression

The art therapist will see a wide range of depressives in any number of different settings. She should keep in mind that not all patients who present a despairing, depressed, dysphoric mode of adjustment come from the same genesis. Depression has different meanings for different people. For some it represents a lack of internalization and loss of meaning, a hunger for direction and mothering on a very basic *pre-symbiotic* level. They need to touch, feel, and sense a caring, understanding therapist. The utilization of a range of sensory materials is a beginning requirement to any work in this area. Essentially, the art therapist builds the world of imagination and feeling. She likewise connects the body with material and experiences and offers a whole range of developmental tasks to aid in the construction of a new being, a new self, and an ego that relates to both the inside and outside. There is also an emphasis on emotional feeding and giving as the art therapist acts as a very primary maternal agent.

Not all depression stems from this genesis. Some depressives are caught in a symbiotic bind of dependency, hate, distrust, and need for autonomy. These depressives are tied within an introjective battle that gives them no peace or freedom. Hate and love fuse while separation anxiety causes an inability to reach out to the present. These patients engage the art therapist in a symbiotic relationship where it is necessary to avoid being induced into the role of the introject. The therapist aids separation and individuation by being with the patient and withstanding fits of rage, anxiety and loss. Materials solidify this encounter by making minimal verbal demands on the patient. Techniques are introduced with an attitude of acceptance and understanding. An implicit statement is constantly made: "I am available, I am with you, I will listen but not take over."

There are still other forms of depression. Some represent a feeling of helplessness when defenses have *decompensated* with accompanying feelings of impotency. Here the art therapist uses her materials to externalize conflicts and provide a field for alternative solutions. As patients test out conflicts in a safe atmosphere, a sense of mastery grows and the depression abates.

Depression can be seen in the whole range of neurotic, characterological, borderline, and psychotic formations. Patients who function near the *schizoid* level need distance rather than feeding. Their emptiness arises from a sense of being eaten up by life. The world is perceived as invading. Art offers distance and opportunities to discover oneself. Materials and stimulants, in these instances, should not be very demanding. The schizoid patient, emptied by forces within and without, needs room to find his own space, as contrasted to others who require constant support. Superficially, these depressed patients may look the same, but the internal dynamics, as well as the application of the art therapy technique, are different. The art therapist can often make the distinction by being very pragmatic in her work. For example, she might ask if feeding brings about a flowing or produces further regression (9).

Character Disorders

A patient with a character disorder typically has an orientation of manipulation, contempt, and a preoccupation with power. The world is perceived as a battleground for action and self-aggrandizement. Character formations take different forms. They range from the explosive acting-out to the passive-aggressive, placative and self-abnegative. The therapeutic problem, however, remains the same—breaking through the character armor, engaging the patient in a real confrontation and overcoming game playing. Thus, there is a need to be very direct as well as knowledgeable of what is happening on a dynamic level in the relationship. All too often art therapists have been "had"; art supplies have been squandered and exploited; the art therapist has been sucked in and used in the service of manipulation which only aids and abets the self-contempt of the patient and reinforces the fantasy of control and power. Thus, the practitioner must use materials judiciously and deal with action and counteraction. Media and techniques that particularly highlight action are very important. What better way is there to confront an acting-out patient than through tape, video, or film? The evidence cannot be denied or dissociated; his behavior is recorded for a return observation. Art and dramatization can help to break through defenses.

At times, this is not enough. Behind these chronic disturbances are deep wells of emptiness and loneliness that are the hallmark of a lack of primary identification and internalization. The therapist must not only be able to present structure and firmness in the relationship, but also care and concern, which facilitate the identification process. As a consequence, the art therapist must be a very touchable and available professional. The authenticity of the therapeutic engagement is an intrinsic part of this process.

As we have reviewed the major diagnostic entities, an important qualification needs constant reiteration: Treatment cannot be approached by thumbing through a diagnostic manual. Dynamics and defenses flow from one level to another. No one patient falls strictly into any one group. A patient who at first seemed a dull plodding obsessive can suddenly develop hysterical symptomatology or perhaps regress to a schizoid solution. The best one can do is to be completely present for a patient, feeling the impact of the relationship, and discovering the uniqueness of each individual's style of life. As the art therapist accrues a clinical frame of experience, she shifts from level to level, integrating the analytic and creative spheres of perception and perspective. Thus, the art therapist loses control, lets something happen, feels the impact of the experience, and slowly puts everything together within a clinical framework. Involved in each contact is the expansion of each individual's creative sphere so that a flow of energy from the cosmic to the adaptational breathes new life in therapeutic endeavors (10, 11).

References

1. Birch, H. *Brain Damage in Children*. Baltimore: Williams and Wilkins, 1964.
2. Evan, T. W. *Brain Injured Children*. Springfield, Illinois: Charles C Thomas, 1969.
3. Saunders, R. J. *Art for the Mentally Retarded in Connecticut*. Hartford, Connecticut: Connecticut State Department of Education, 1967.
4. Levin, S. and Kabana, R. *Psychodynamic Studies on Aging—Creativity, Reminiscing and Dying*. New York: International Universities Press, 1967.
5. Searles, H. *Collected Papers on Schizophrenia*. New York: International Universities Press, 1965.
6. Burton, W. *Psychotherapy of the Psychosis*. New York: Basic Books, 1961.
7. Fenichel, O. *The Psychodynamic Theory of Neurosis*. New York: W. W. Norton, 1945.

8. Kubie, L. S. *Neurotic Distortion of the Creative Process.* New York: Noonday Press, 1961.

9. Greenacre, P. *Affective Disorders.* New York: International Universities Press, 1953.

10. Redl, F. and Wineman, D. *Controls from Within.* Glencoe, Illinois: Free Press, 1952.

11. Reich, W. *Character Analysis.* New York: Orgone Institute Press, 1949.

8. Institutional Issues

Art therapy cannot be taught in a vacuum. Becoming a professional entails a pragmatic exposure to the realities of practice. With field-work, the importance of the political nature of institutions and the impact it has on treatment become paramount issues for the art therapy intern. Theory, by necessity, is modified by the limitations of the agency structure (1).

Health care institutions are flooded with patients. There is simply not enough staff, space, time or funds to adequately cope with the multitude of problems. Consequently, a change may soon occur: The anxious, idealistic and enthusiastic student transforms into a depressed, despairing and bewildered practitioner. She wonders if anything can be done, what functions she serves and what she can accomplish. The student recognizes slowly that she must understand the political realities of the institution in order to work with patients. One cannot function in isolation. The institution ultimately determines an atmosphere that has tremendous impact on the direction of treatment. If the setting is uncaring, concerned only with statistics and disconnected in its overall administrative procedures, then this tone undoubtedly will affect the therapist-patient relationship. As a result the student's education must be broadened to include a psychological understanding of the institution as a political entity.

An institution can be approached like a patient. Some are restricted and tight; others are disorganized and even schizophrenic! At times they are disconnected, destructive, vague and fragmented. Occasionally, an institution works in coordinated teams with cohesiveness and unity. Unfortunately, the latter rarely happens. Professionals have grave difficulties in maintaining sanity and identity when they find themselves in an essentially pathological setting. To withdraw, to be embittered or to be frustrated is understandable but does nothing to change the situation. To be uninvolved with institutional politics does not serve patients and destroys the student's personal and professional effectiveness. The art therapist simply cannot cop out and expect to survive in the field.

Like a patient, an institution brings distortions, inductions, projections, and "double-bind" communications. These forces need to be recognized, attended and confronted. But as with a patient, the art therapist must first develop rapport with her co-workers before anything can be done. For instance, the art therapist who starts out in an occupational therapy department can be requested to supervise patients in nonimaginative tasks. Art therapists resent this; they are threatened and sometimes react openly with anger. Routine, repetitive work seems antithetical to the whole concept of art therapy. Nevertheless, a therapist needs to understand that art has long been used for this purpose. Consequently, the student soon learns how to respond to the institution's notion of art therapy and to include other concepts, such as problem-solving, that relate to other levels and goals of the agency. Thus, art can be used as a way to increase ego capacities, facilitate mastery over problem situations, and become the format to develop socialization skills. Again, as in the therapeutic relationship, the application of these concepts meets the institution on a comprehensible level. If, on the other hand, the student acts out with negativism or hostility, she will be unable to develop a mutual base of operations where the administrative perception of her role can change gradually. Large organizations take years to develop: Personnel structures, communications systems, procedures and operational patterns each have a genesis and purpose. The art therapy intern cannot naively approach complex institutional problems, expecting overnight change, any more than she would expect a chronic schizophrenic to deal effectively with reality after one semester of treatment. Organizations thrive on homeostasis. They resent and fight change; people do not want their own positions within the structure jeopardized. The art therapy student represents an unknown quantity. Though she often begins at the bottom of the totem pole, because of her training, talents and skills, she poses a potential threat to the security needs of others.

Agencies are expected to be mothering and caring agents. Often, however, settings are equally perceived as overwhelming, dominating, or engulfing. If the intern selectively hooks countertransference problems on pieces of the institutional reality, this will only interfere with her effectiveness. The handling of induced reactions caused by institutional pressures is as sensitive and demanding a task as any found in depth psychotherapy. Personal therapy and membership in peer discussion groups, as well as other professional associations, are needed to maintain some degree of sanity and perspective.

Clarity and specificity provide important guidelines to follow in dealing with organizations. For instance, training institutes should insist on very clear and concise affiliation contracts for their students. The clarification of obligations, responsibilities, and duties of the field and training institutions, as well as of the particular student, helps to avoid potential obstacles. Hours, working conditions, type of supervision, and the insistence on professional treatment can initiate a working foundation from the beginning. Art therapists can be helped by an awareness of the institution's tendency to reinforce a sense of malaise and stagnation. Professionals grow all too comfortable in their roles, causing a lack of inventiveness, risk-taking and growth. One remedy might be continued training outside the setting. The therapist can also be open to exploration of new avenues and definitions for her work. Initiating help from professionals outside one's baliwick can be the beginning of a rich cross fertilization process. A concrete example would be the art therapist who functions in a primarily medical and surgical unit. Along with medical, nursing, liaison psychiatric, teaching and social work staff, she can suggest an interdisciplinary team geared to understanding patient and staff realities from all perspectives.

The effectiveness of an art therapy trainee can be enhanced by a sensitive understanding of the institution's communication network. Administrative lines of responsibility, format for memos, and time lapses all form part of this knowledge. This network may impair as well as facilitate effective communication. Red tape! Memos and requisitions are written, lost, ignored and filed, often bogged down at one level or another. Even more frustrating is the difficulty of determining responsibility for the resistance and reason for institutional buck-passing. Avoidance of decision-making is also a common phenomenon. An art therapist studying this network will learn to use it to her best advantage, since change necessitates knowledge of the ins and outs of an administrative structure. Patience and persistance sometimes stimulate this process and effect change. If the intern gives up easily, the institution will wear her down to a state of despair and stagnation.

Art therapy cannot be divorced from the economic problems that beset health care institutions. Each department has a vested interest in obtaining a share of limited space and funds, and, of necessity, an administrator's main concern is getting the most productivity for his money. Art therapy may be considered a luxury in this respect. A good deal of education and clarification can change this perception. A patient's increased functioning can often be a direct result of increased emotional health. For instance, art therapy on a pediatric unit may have a profound impact on preparation for surgery, remission and post-hospitalization adjustment (2). Creative play in educational settings may directly affect reading and achievement scores (3). The time for rehabilitation of psychiatric patients can be cut with the use of art therapy treatment (4). There is not, however, a clear and obvious relationship between art therapy and increased performance and, therefore, optimum use of funds. The most powerful way to establish causality and substantiate opinion is a wealth of research bringing objectivity and perspective to this problem.

Agencies rarely have a position or "line" for an art therapist. Consequently, students are often assigned to the occupational or recreational therapy department. On occasion, the intern is expected to function as a mother's helper who can keep the patients busy and, only incidentally, offer a therapeutic art experience. Rarely is there any sense of the training, perspective, philosophy and orientation of the art therapist. More often, a good deal of confusion between art and occupational therapy exists. The art therapist cannot immediately change these preconceived attitudes. Patience and a development of trust between the individual art therapist and other professionals are indispensable and can only be affected through constant communication and mutual sharing of experiences. Politically, art therapists need supportive friends. Hopefully, they will search for staff sympathetic to change and innovation. Exhibits, fairs and case presentations are some of the communicative skills of the intern. She can also learn the verbiage or professional nomenclature of the organization and revitalize the words and labels so they take on new meaning that is comprehensible and mutual. For example, instead of recounting a patient's play experience, one might invite other professionals at a staff meeting to become involved with art media.

Art therapists need not segregate themselves from other expressive therapists. All forms of expression can and should be used with any one patient or group of patients. Departmental divisions of dance, music and art seem artificial and at times politicized. The art therapist should be ready to share her skills with other expressive therapists and

learn from them. It is hoped that she can communicate a degree of
mutuality and cooperation in sharing and working with other closely
aligned professionals.

Art therapists who work in school systems are sometimes experienced as a threat to the territorial prerogatives of psychologists and
guidance personnel. The latter need to hear that art therapy presents
an added dimension to children who do not have the verbal tools
to work in the more standardized fashion. Constant study and research
are needed here also as a connecting link between creativity development and the mastery of basic skills. Art therapists who are unaware
or uninvolved with the goals of the educational institution may be
stymied in their attempts to initiate art therapy in schools. The
trainee, therefore, must have a very clear theoretical model of the
relationship among sensory awareness, imagery production, and conceptual thinking. Frontiers in the use of art therapy in schools are
currently being explored. To go further, the student may need to
incorporate adaptive and creative expression into an operational framework that makes sense to an educator, such as combining remedial
reading with art therapy.

Similar principles should be maintained in other institutional settings. Art therapy can be combined with vocational guidance and
rehabilitation procedures. Fantasy play can develop into an exploration
of the world of work, by, for example, setting up creative play situations
to test out work skills. In day care centers, tactile, expressive and imaginative techniques can be employed to solve the problems of separation,
growth and mastery. Old age and nursing homes need the artist as
an ally to combat loneliness and boredom as well as to find a tool to
help put life in order. In all of these examples, the young professional
must sense the aim of the institution and fit her particular skills into
a facilitation and implementation of the agency's mission.

In some settings, the intern may find encounter techniques employed by poorly trained staff resulting in sadism, exploitation and
abuse of patients. If the art therapist chooses to work with groups,
she can not always identify or prevent this but needs to constantly
search for therapeutic models based on knowledge and sophistication.
The student may well have to demonstrate the important difference
between toughness or firmness and out-and-out cruelty. Support from
other staff members who are sympathetic to these values will help
immeasurably in maintaining one's integrity.

An art therapist who can relate not only to the interpersonal dynamics of the setting but to the ecological factors as well will offer a unique asset to her agency. Enhancing the mood and the rhythm of the institution can affect the well-being of patients as well as staff. Changing the psychic, spatial and color world of patients may be a most challenging dimension of the art therapist's role. The somber walls of a ward can use colorful creative products for the benefit of both patient and staff. In addition, staff are also made aware of creative energies. Emotional growth and learning cannot be separated from the physical spatial attributes.

Art therapists may need to band together to form their own institutions as a viable alternative to the existing agency structure. These particular ventures, however idealistically based, are fraught with difficulties and pressures. Professionals who take this alternative should be prepared to clearly work through their purpose and function. Economic pressures will be immense and a familiarity with funding procedures is indispensable. A part-time affiliation with an institution may be essential, if only to maintain a monetary flow for survival.

In summary, the art therapist must have a sensitive understanding of and educated response to the prevailing political realities of a particular agency setting. In a particular setting, the budding intern may find herself fitting more into the model of social catalyst rather than therapist. She may also learn to flex and stretch her professional skills so that she can move out to settings that are somewhat atypical. Storefronts, parks and clubhouses are potential places for an art therapist to effect social change and facilitate creative movement through art. The art therapist, therefore, is not linked to one image or notion of community involvement but is able to discover new and different settings where her work can be appreciated and her personal goals fulfilled.

Working in most institutions is no easy task. Until we find a better way to deal with the problems of society, institutions are here to stay with their attendant ills, problems, and peculiarities. Hopefully, the creativity of the art therapist will stand her in good stead when she confronts the stagnation and oppression of agency work. In spite of all these obstacles, it is important to note that patients *do* get help; organizations *do* change; new professions *are* emerging and the art therapist is finding ever-increasing opportunities to become an effective professional. During the past five years, the opportunities for work as an art therapist in the New York area alone have increased dramatically (5).

Something seems to be happening and changing. We are often so submerged in the morass of obstacles and pressures that it is difficult to maintain perspective and observe the process of institutional growth. Somewhere the idealism of the new student faced with political realities does cope with her despair and confusion. Out of this experience she creates a pragmatic approach, supported by hope, vision and flexibility and sustained by a large supply of energy.

References

1. Dumont, P. *The Absurd Healer: Perspectives of a Community Psychiatrist.* New York: Science House, 1968.
2. Le Grand, D. D. "Psychoanalytic Principles Applied to Pediatric Surgery." *Maryland State Medical Journal,* 113–117, March, 1964.
3. Linderman, E. W. and Herberholz, D. W. *Developing Artistic and Perceptual Awareness: Art Practice in the Elementary Classroom.* 2nd ed. Dubuque, Iowa: W. C. Brown, 1969.
4. Result of interview with Phyllis Miller, A.T.R., Director, Day Hospital, Mt. Sinai Medical Center, New York.
5. Based on survey of Pratt Institute field placement records 1971–1975.

II. CASE STUDIES

9. Art Psychotherapy: Four Perspectives

Linda Beth Sibley, "Deanna," Arthur Robbins and Gilbert L. Gordon

The following case study is presented in four segments: the first part describing the relationship from the therapist's perspective was written by Linda Beth Sibley, M.P.S., A.T.R. Deanna (a pseudonym), the patient, then describes her version of the experience. The third and fourth segments give the reader the opportunity to understand the art therapy process from two points of view: Arthur Robbins, Ed.D., A.T.R., is a Freudian analyst on the faculty of the National Psychological Association for Psychoanalysis, and Gilbert L. Gordon, M.D. is a Jungian oriented psychoanalyst.

THE ART THERAPIST'S VIEWPOINT

I see Deanna in my studio for art therapy as an adjunct to her Jungian analysis. Her analyst, B., enthusiastically recommended her to me after I had several meetings with him and had expressed a desire to practice art therapy and explore how creativity could contribute to growth in the analytic relationship. D. is 31 years old and has been in analysis for about six months when we begin our work together. She is married to a banker, R., and has two children—a boy, six, and a girl, four years old. An attractive woman, she is tall and large, 150 lbs. Her concern over her appearance focuses on her losing weight and the sophistication of her clothes. D. has been a grade school teacher but is currently working as a secretary to several college professors. Her parents are both alive and live in the suburbs. D. comes to the loft once a week for two hours. Her label would probably be "healthy neurotic"; she is seeking to make confluent her inner and outer realities, to find out what she feels and believes about herself and act upon those feelings to direct her life.

When we began working, D. described a disturbing incongruity between her rich fantasy life, dreams and wishes and the reality of her life situation. B., her analyst, was her best friend, more understanding than her husband, and he was helping her deal with past and present material. She has a strong need for a female confidante and I have stepped into that role, among others. D.'s commitment to our work together was shaky at first but has increased; although she is moving to the suburbs soon, she plans to come into the city and continue working with B. and myself.

I had two contradictory feelings at the beginning of my relationship with D.: excitement and fear. I returned from the arts and therapy conference in England, enthusiasm overflowing to begin analytic work with patients. I had known B. for several years and looked forward to learning from him and sharing my art perspective. My fear took hold when I realized I had not previously presented myself as a professional for another adult to experience and judge. I gained security from the environment, my home, and by allowing D. to pay me only $5 per hour—I was a beginner and really couldn't be worth much more. My anxiety, along with D.'s, caused our initial interactions to be on a rather superficial level. We began each session with a cup of coffee; it was informal, gave each of us an object to focus on and represented nourishment—something we were both after. D. was excellent at avoiding serious discussion and relieving her anxiety by flooding me with verbal information. I allowed this for a while for several reasons—my own fear (of what?), respect of her defenses, and my perception that she was not ready for greater involvement (or was she just fooling me?). Gradually I broke through her manipulation by following my instincts with either art exercises or role-playing. Later D. referred to these specific instances as the most valuable for her. I broke through the overwhelming verbiage mostly because it bored me; my mind wandered and I yawned. I have a strong feeling that the crucial timing of a push was based on my intuition—unconscious— and not just a conscious impatience. At times I felt very unconnected to her—close but not intimate. At other times I felt numbed and professionally distanced. Building our connection to one another has been slow but is increasing presently. The real links consist of the clay work, D.'s mandalas and our work together of sculpting and casting a portrait bust of her father. It has been the art work that was the catalyst that cut through the tendency in both of us to give in to fear and intellectual nonsense chatter.

The Role of Deanna's Analyst

B., D.'s analyst, and I conferred about once a month. The initial goals he suggested to me were to allow D.: 1) to choose and follow through on a project (she has great difficulty making decisions and has interests in a myriad of directions); and 2) to improve her body image. As our work progressed the emphasis shifted to offering the listening, attentive support of a woman friend and to increase her feeling of self-worth by accomplishments in art media. The project of sculpting a bust of her father was companion work to D.'s work with B. on understanding this relationship through dreams, experiences and feelings. It is difficult to explain whether D. set goals for B. and me or we for her; they evolved among us. This was most clearly evident in the father-daughter situation; all three of us could relate to the archetype. There was less repetition and competition among us than I might have expected.

Movement

The flow of our involvement—what we have created together—has had three distinct phases. Our dance began with D.'s missing the first session; she was apologetic and I was disappointed and relieved. She compensated for this by bringing me a dream and illustrating it the next week. This avoidance/contact rhythm became a pattern. Coffee, cigarettes, chatter, my painting and the radio music, chatter, gum chewing and Ann Landers questions, and chatter, chatter, chatter. I yawned and my mind wandered; I felt frustrated and reached to touch her. She put me off and then accused, "Why did you let me get away with that?" Dancing back and forth and a little art work near the end to ease both our consciences. We changed manipulator and manipulated, were very anxious, learning to trust each other and fearing rejection and failure. I tried Gestalt techniques and failed for they were not me and I was not using my own power. Next there seemed to be some sort of trust and a complete abandonment of the psychological structure which neither of us was comfortable with and an involvement in the art work. We would have coffee and talk—but only to calm each other's anxiety—for about 15–20 minutes and then two hours-plus of hard work would follow. Conversation continued but was definitely secondary to the act of creation. Our mutual excitement was inspiring; we fed each other. I felt a little guilty at not getting to "feelings" but more strongly "right" in following my instincts that what we were doing was what we both needed to do. It felt solid and good; D. rekindled some of my creative energy and I began to work on my own. We were both drawing mandalas. We connected clearly and a caring began. Phase three has been the casting of the clay model and is characterized by a good deal less tension, less urgency, greater ease and depth of discussion, facing of real issues and less chatter. Both of us seem to be more perceptive. I am teacher and D. student, but casting cannot be done alone and requires smooth teamwork.

Individually, D. began our work at the tail end of a long plateau of confusion, depression, indecision, being off center. In four months she has changed markedly, making the statement, "I feel so good, there's nothing I couldn't handle." I hope the feeling lasts. My own process has been almost diametrically opposed to D.'s. Though we have certainly influenced each other, the forces contributing to these changes have been, I believe, more outside our relationship than a result of it. If the movement were the melody, perhaps the issues we discussed will provide the harmony. I realize that they are subjects more than contents but do believe that they are necessary for a complete portrait.

Issues

D.'s first statements at our initial meeting were, "I'm depressed. I have gained weight and I'm hungry." She came to see me directly after Weight Watchers and always reported on her progress upon entering. Nourishment in the form of food was gradually replaced, a little by her work with B. and me, and by her own ability to psychically feed herself. Food has continued to crop up in our talks until near the end of therapy. Clay forms and crayon drawings always seem to remind her of specific dishes, she asked for recipes and my diet and how I stayed slim, etc. We talked of her figure; she is terribly self-conscious but knows how to dress to disguise her size. She perceives herself as a fat child and longs to be slim and beautiful and sophisticated. I perceive her as a large attractive woman trying to become what she is not and bewildered by the frustration. I was surprised at her weight; I do not think of her as heavy or fat. She encumbers herself only by denying her self-psyche and soma—for an illusion.

A second aspect of her illusion is her love of New York City, and the excitement and sophistication it represents. D. is an extrovert and not at all satisfied with the limitations of her role as wife and mother. She yearns to be a career woman, to have a stimulating social life, to take lessons and improve herself and attend lectures and concerts. In this respect, the collective feelings of women in this country can be seen manifested in D. R., her husband, is an introvert, like myself, and content to stay at home and collect stamps. She loves him dearly but sometimes finds him boring. D. personifies her frustration at being limited by her family and her guilt about desiring a life outside the home by a love of "the city." She rarely takes advantage of cultural events and until recently would not socialize without R.

D. continually has expressed dissatisfaction with her job as a secretary (not the right image) and talked of returning to teaching as a more interesting alternative. She was fired as a teacher several years ago but seems to have confidence in her abilities. Though she has gone to a few interviews, she hasn't really pushed. There are too many other possibilities that might be more rewarding and she can't bring herself to make a decision.

An inability to choose and follow through is evident in her attempts at self-improvement—singing, acting, art, writing—and also in pursuing job possibilities—teaching, real estate. The pattern was broken in our work by a contract. D. chose a project, the sculpture. The process is long and arduous; at this writing we have spent five weeks and have at least three to go. Several sessions have been four or five hours long. She did not back out of the situation but rather worked enthusiastically the whole time. Perhaps she needed a partner and I filled the bill. When complete, she will have a physical manifestation of her ability to choose, create and complete a project.

Intimacy is the real knot around which D's problems revolve. She is aware of it as an issue with women much more clearly than with men. D. regularly speaks of not having a close female friend; her last "best friend" always thought that whatever D. said or did was "great—fantastic." Fortunately or unfortunately, she moved to South America for six years. I have replaced her on one level. Transference was tested by D. as she repeated her comment often to see if I would really be able to offer her the all-accepting support and love she needed. My hope is that I have offered it—but in my way—not the friend's. I am an attentive listener; I keep her secrets, respect her defenses, encourage her attempts at growth and do not criticize her behavior. I also hope I have responded honestly when she has sought my opinions. The friend was somehow wonderful but beneath D.; I am more an equal and a puzzle. At times she wonders how I can have it "all together" and be six years younger than she. This feeling is expressed by a mixed admiration and jealousy for my "generation": 1) I didn't accept parental values and marry and bear children before I realized more of my own potential as an individual; and 2) though I do have a beau, I could sleep around if I wanted to. I have recently tried to use our intimacy to destroy a few of D.'s illusions and explain honestly my experience of facing these questions: Life—it's all the same whether you are 31 or 25. Personal awareness and strength are not a result of your date of birth. My own feelings beyond that are confused but the discussion of a safe impersonal topic such as this seems to be the way D. begins to define her own feelings.

To return to intimacy, D. feels much closer to her daughter than to her son, to her mother than her father; this is not unusual but it is important when regarded alongside the question of intimacy with men, beginning with her father, her husband and other men. At our third meeting we discussed A, B and C people, A people being the most important and close, having the qualities of acceptance, trust and love. D. said she couldn't express her feelings freely with A people. Her analyst was the only exception and he was more her best friend than her husband. An inability to communicate with her parents, particularly her father, had always been a problem. Her father continually surprises her because she doesn't know him at all. They either avoid each other or sit in the same room and do not speak. D. feels caring and love but cannot give it to or receive it from him.

Her father and husband have the same name. She "respects and admires and loves" her husband but cannot talk with him honestly about her confusion nor her desires to develop herself outside the family setting. There is a silent space between them that has been building for the duration of their marriage, and is only recently being destroyed and replaced by a mutual openness and tolerance of the individual process. This space has existed to a certain degree because of D.'s need to have sexual relations with other men. R. may be aware of this—D. thinks not, but she cannot bring herself to tell him. B. feels that D. is wise in this respect; R. has not been at a point to accept this information and a marriage that does have value and substance and is worth maintaining could be lost.

D. sees her affairs as part of the image of an exciting urban woman. She feels some guilt but not a sufficient amount to cease the pattern of behavior. She feels her lovers provide fun, intrigue and intimacy that she is missing in the rest of her life. They mean enough for her to lie to her husband and to cancel one of our dates together. D. seemed to have missed part of the adolescent stage of development and married early one of her first loves. She never had the sexual freedom she envies so in my generation. D. chooses men that are good material for fantasy but in reality unavailable for anything other than affairs. They have the characteristics she feels deficient in herself—intelligence, charm, savoir faire, independence and good looks.

While we have been together D. has had one affair. She mentioned K. at our third session and disclosed a more complete story during our next meeting. I think the rapid intimacy between us was partially a result of her need for a confidante. I listened and said little; D. did not want judgments, just air time. I felt uncomfortable partially because I did not feel close enough with her for such a confession—it seemed like such explosive material. I was resentful and confused by the topic. The level of D.'s sexual interpersonal relationships seemed something I had outgrown in college. She thought sexuality was intimacy; she could only be close with men if she were in bed. B. was her first male friend; they have spent some time working on this confusion and still are. I became alternately fascinated and impatient; a woman who was 31 years old had a part of her that was 17 and it was controlling her life to some extent. She had missed an experience that is so important to me—having close friends who are men. D. was aware of certain projections she made concerning K. The affair ended after several weeks. Both of us needed to understand the meaning of her behavior and individually talked with B. Once the affair ended, D. never mentioned it to me again.

B.'s theory of a possible understanding of D.'s affair was explained in Jung's terminology. Although some of these are his thoughts, upon rereading my own notes of D.'s feelings, they seem appropriate. As my work with D. progresses it further substantiates B.'s interpretation (patient fitting therapist's philosophical framework?).

D.'s parents lack good feeling communication between themselves and with their children. D.'s Mom was always critical of her, made her feel worthless and "like shit," the ugly, fat, little girl. Mom never affirmed a positive feminine image by her behavior or in D.; Dad was very fond of D. and emotionally tied to her, perhaps as an opportunity for psychic intimacy he lacked with his wife. D. then appeared a threat to the parental union, symbolizing potential incest (psychic in this culture), and was rejected by both parents. The aggressive animus mother stood between the father and daughter and prohibited any close relationship. To Dad she became a subject too explosive to become involved with and he cut off all feelings. The parents switched roles—Mom/aggressive/animus and Dad/passive/anima. D. now carries the weight of all the unexpressed feelings as well as the tension caused by the role reversal. She has become a threat to both her parents partially as a result of everyone's inability to release emotionally laden impulses (1).

D. has had little affirmation of her feminine self from either parent, brother or husband. D. was R.'s first love and he was not particularly experienced with women. She has a void of feminine feelings about herself as a woman of relatedness, which she responds to by trying to fill it the only way she knows—sexually—thereby fulfilling the incest archetype. While the feminine remains underdeveloped, the animus grows in power; D. does come on very strong. The animus as a woman's light bearer finds an excellent example in D. (2). He throws light on so many interests and possibilities that she can never make a decision. He is out of her control much of the time.

D., only now becoming aware of her family dynamics, is moving in two directions. One is to begin opening her relationship with her husband. More and more she honestly communicates her desires to him. They have read *Open Marriage* (3) and started to change their life-style. Honesty became important when they made a decision to buy a house and move from the city. Before making the commitment and signing the contract, D. made it clear that she loved R. and would move to the country if he was aware of her intention to fully live her own life and pursue interests outside the family. To her surprise, R. offered no resistance. She had expected disapproval, and still does before each encounter, since she had met with disapproval from R. in the past and from her father. R. is also growing and changing. My guess is that if D. personifies his unconscious, he too would like to explore new interests and possibilities within himself. Perhaps he will absorb some of her strength, curiosity and sense of adventure. D. is finding R.'s stay-at-home routine more palatable as the other parts of her self are allowed expression.

The second move is in the direction of her Dad. At Christmas D. made special efforts with just the right gifts and warm conversation to reopen her lines of communication with her father; she was very successful and amazed at her own power. In our work, she chose to sculpt her Dad, not her husband or children, and has spent about 20 hours, great care and love to make it very special. He was deeply touched at learning of the project.

My feelings about D.'s father anima/animus problem are not clear; I'm blocking a lot because the feelings have relevance. My father (who synchronistically just telephoned for the first time in six months) and I are also unrelated. We communicate far better by letter than in person. There is no question of love—it's there—but expression is restricted by a void similar to D's. Though our situations have likenesses, I do not intend to take on D.'s psychic burdens for my own. I have thought a lot about my father as a result of D. Perhaps I can follow her courage in dealing with an explosive situation.

Art

At our first meeting D. did a cake box (Figures 9.1 and 9.2, see Color Illustrations, p. D), an Elaine Rapp technique (4). I asked her to illustrate her perception of how others see her on the outside of the box and her perception of herself on the inside. She could then put it together as a paper sculpture or a box, any way she chose. Figure 9.1 is a plan of her apartment. R. and the kids are drawn but not D. She resonated strongly with the kitchen (nourishment) window (perception) hung with growing plants and guarded by an iron railing ("to keep out rats"). Figure 9.2 illustrates a dream she had the night before. It moves from bottom to top: D.'s hand is shown reaching for a red balloon. The balloon has a Bozo the Clown nose, is marked 7D and rings like a telephone. She follows its beckoning ring into the dark stairwell of an apartment building. A strange and sinister man rushes past and she gets out of his way. D. talks into the intercom and tells the voice she will not walk up seven flights. D. goes outside and it is dusk. A warm and friendly policeman takes her arm and they stroll the promenade under street lamps and trees casting shadows. It is very pleasant and she feels no fear. The man has a gentle, appealing face which D. takes care to depict.

We talked some of her lack of a body attached to the hand and face or distinct figure in the third part. The dream analysis she did with B. My own associations for the three stages (Greek) of D.'s dream are: 1. Play, child, follow, communication; 2. unrelated man, bad father, danger, animus; 3. related man, good animus, authority. My guess as to the meaning can only be: Follow the play (toy) and experience the bad and, finally, good masculine parts of D.'s self. I'm sure there is more—but D. didn't share the information. It was our first encounter and I respected her privacy. As an initial dream it certainly pointed out where we would eventually find our work together.

D. next made a pinch pot (Figure 3, see Color Illustration, p. E) which she wanted tall and skinny and came out short and fat. It has a pie crust rim and brought her minimal satisfaction. Figure 9.4 (see Color Illustration, p. E) shows two waves. This was made in response to my request that she give form to her feelings of simultaneous joy and sadness. I asked her to become the wave. Her monologue went something like this: "I am a wave and feel joy at riding high and bubbling and curling around. I am beautiful and clear and glassy. I glide and undulate and crash! On the shore I ebb and flow and feel sad at being pulled out to sea."

This was the first time we really connected. D.'s last comment the previous week was how her parents and relatives thought she was crazy. After her monologue I asked her if she could share these feelings with her parents. She said no. She couldn't tell them in fantasy, in an empty chair or if I played Mom or Dad. I trusted my unconscious and pushed and asked D. if I could speak for her. I did, being gentle but honest and trying to repeat her words. "Mom, I feel happy and sad and want to share this with you. But I can't. You make me feel small and worthless and it hurts me. I know you don't mean to be thought-less but please be more aware. I am worthwhile and I know it. You love R. and the kids but not me. Try harder, I know you can." Very heavy. D. cried. I panicked at what I had done. I broke the tension after a minute with tissues and some humor. D. later told me how meaningful it had been to her. I trusted my instincts; I had no con-scious awareness or control of what I was doing. Very dangerous, I thought, but I was lucky. I didn't understand at the time how I had plugged into those feelings since I couldn't identify them with my mother at all—but I could with my father and that intuition proved to be more correct than I guessed.

Figure 9.5 (see Color Illustration, p. E) is a family of slab pots, "like B. has on his desk." D., surprised at her ability, is beginning to sense her own creative power. No particular discussion was connected with these other than D.'s comment that her first pot had a big hole in it. They can be seen as her family unit or as the four functions: sensation, feeling, intuition and thinking.

Figures 9.6 through 9.11 (see Color Illustrations, pp. F–G) are a series of mandalas D. began at my suggestion after having met Joan Kellogg in Columbus, Ohio. They are numbered in sequence and were executed at the end of each session (all are done in cray pas on 14" x 18" paper). They do tell a characteristic something of our encounters and are always drawn to the left (unconscious) side of the page (5).

Deanna begins with a sad and depressed woman, crying through her emphatic smile (Figure 9.6). The tears cannot be held within the circle and run down her face, past radiating yellow and blue energy suggesting either the sun and/or barbs that protect her vulnerability. The second mandala (Figure 9.7), a snail, shows an increasing curiosity and engagement in our process. D. said, "Everything seems so difficult, but when I start in the center and follow my path—it all becomes so simple. I just had to continue out, beyond the limit." The snail's antennae are repeated in the stamen of the only blooming flower in the next mandala (Figure 9.8). The earth colors of browns, green and yellow are used to draw the seedlings, portraying some force moving and growing—and almost in bloom.

Somehow the fourth mandala (Figure 9.9) was a puzzle to us both: It seemed unlike the three previous organic forms. The colors were opposite, pink and green, the design suggested mountains and valleys, M for man and W for woman—all opposites creating tension within a circumference that was reinforced three times. All the energy contained within this mandala explodes in the next magic circle (Figure 9.10)—surely magic for it clearly proclaims D.'s new sense of being, self-assurance and joy. The colors in the top half are those of the rainbow (foreseen in the tears and sunlight of Figure 9.6). The bottom half was left empty ". . . for room to grow, for something unknown." This split did not disturb either of us, we were so elated over our surplus of good feeling about ourselves and our work.

The last mandala (Figure 9.11) resembles a pink and red chrysanthemum in full bloom. It has a reinforced central design that lies slightly askew. The circles and arcs reminded me of an early American quilt pattern called the double wedding ring. D. denied any intention at all, claiming it flowed rhythmically through her hand onto the paper. As the sixth mandala, it fulfills the seedling in the third drawing and completes the series.

While the mandalas provide a kind of record, they also represent a technique D. has integrated as a way of getting in touch with her own power. I suggested that she draw mandalas at home whenever she felt off center or out of control. Though I haven't seen them, she tells me she has drawn several—some at home and some at her parents' over the holidays when she became overwhelmed by family and relatives. I tune into the centered and whole qualities; D. said they gave her a reassurance of her own worth and a sense of power after her Mom had been particularly insensitive. To me, that's what art therapy and creativity development are all about. When I was depressed D. told me to use my own medicine and by golly, it works! While drawing a mandala I have felt the tension leave my body and somehow have been filled up or re-inspirited and able to return to my studies.

Figure 9.12 (see Color Illustration, p. H) shows the clay bust of D.'s Dad before casting. D. once remarked that I wouldn't believe the extent of her fantasy life. When she tried to stall the actual beginning of the sculpture, I asked her to fantasize herself as a sculptress—and make the fantasy come alive, now! We worked together in the beginning but only D. worked as the clay became a person. It began as a boy and grew to a man and then Spencer Tracy and then an older man and then Dad. For two sessions she thought of it as R., and not her Dad, until we gave him jowls and a receding hairline. I instructed on anatomy and D. and I both consulted several instamatic photographs constantly. Our involvement was so intense—we were both elated and exhausted by the end of each session, now lasting four or five hours instead of two, but neither of us wanted to stop. D.'s sense of achievement and pride is so exciting. She has tapped a creative source (she's *very* good) that she was unaware of. Our meetings became inspiring and energizing for both of us. I began drawing on my own and felt so good after spending time with her. After our first five-hour workout, before Christmas, we gave each other a big hug. It felt great—the flow of energy was astonishing. D. keeps shouting "I can't believe we did it. It's great; I did that! It *really* looks like him." We laugh and smile a lot and work even harder.

Two issues are raised: 1. Should I have kept my hands off the sculpture more? I got too excited. We talked about it and how I wanted her to feel it was her creation. She said she did and allowed me to touch it only for anatomical reasons—as her teacher. She felt she learned about seeing closely, and about physical anatomy. It was important to clear up this issue between us for us to stay open about each other. 2. How much of my joy at being involved was a relief at legitimately avoiding the therapist role and becoming a teacher or partner? Some. My dream: *I am leading group therapy—D., two women, and my grandmother. Two brothers and a sister are sitting on the side. I am serving liquor and thinking of showing slides of my art work. I am a bad therapist.* My feeling still stands that mutual teaching was what our relationship constellated. We are much more strongly connected by having done something together than by all the chatter-nonsense-talking in the world. Through the art work—and not my junior psychiatry or D.'s dumping verbal garbage—we formed an alliance.

Summary

We have started the third phase I mentioned earlier—more relaxed and flowing, less avoidance by both of us and working right along. We began to discuss Dad for the first time on a deeper level and both discovered new perspectives. The casting is almost complete and the carving and chipping will begin. D.'s father has not been made anew yet—he's imprisoned in two inches of plaster and she must free him.

My feelings about her have changed radically. As our movement went from more talk than art work to more art work than talk, I got to know her. I hope we find a balance. D. was a profession or a project for a while, but now she is closer to a friend. I might not choose her for a friend socially, but I care about her a great deal; it's a new kind of love. Her process and growth touch my heart as well as intriguing my intellectual curiosity. We have learned much from each other.

My questions are all about specific instances rather than dynamics. I would rather let the process happen than talk about it any more. My dream tells me what I should know. Finally, I feel excitement at having completed the assignment; I have learned from myself and D. while I have written. I find greater satisfaction in the time I spend with her than seven times that amount I spend at my institutional fieldwork placement. I also feel fraudulent because there is so much left unsaid—specific instances and pieces to the puzzle, the quality of feeling between us, and, most of all, what our experience together has actually been and meant. However, it cannot be written and I'm not sure something like this should be shared.

I would like to express my warmest thanks to B. for his trust in me, his patience and support in our work together.

DEANNA'S REFLECTIONS

I have always made a very conscious search for meaning in life—something to make my life worthwhile. People have often said that I was talented in this or creative in that area but there was no person or idea or talent to which I was willing to commit my life. Restless and discontented, I could never seem to find satisfaction in any accomplishment or feeling or memory. When things became unbearably boring, my restlessness would manifest itself in a job change or in insisting on moving the family to a new home.

It was when I was approaching 30, was a wife and mother and a teacher, and very busy (always hoping that each new activity would be *the* one to which I could devote myself) that women's liberation, my dislike for teaching (an activity which threatened to consume all my life and time and from which I derived little satisfaction) and my general dissatisfaction with my life made me press for a move to New York City, a place I have always viewed as the most exciting and interesting place on earth.

New York did prove to be an important move for I loved all of it and there were millions of activities and people and jobs to choose from. To make some money, but again without committing myself to a career, I found a secretarial job at a school which, as expected, was boring, but the atmosphere of the school was stimulating and I could take courses free. I chose a course in C. G. Jung's psychology and found it interesting and exciting. The teacher was a Jungian analyst and, the class being small, I got to know him and finally asked him if I could work with him. I was hoping to find through analysis the cause of the restlessness in my life.

One of the most important ideas to come out of those analytic sessions, which were extremely important to me in many ways, was a quotation by my analyst of Dieter Baumann: "Your creativity takes precedence over everything else in your life. If you don't pay attention to your creativity, you will dissolve."

Creativity to me meant art and art meant drawing, painting, sculpting, etc., so when my analyst mentioned that he knew of a young art therapist who wanted to collaborate with him on a project involved with her studies and that because it was her first such case she was willing to see me for a very small fee, I was very eager to begin the search for my creativity with her.

Very soon thereafter I met Linda Sibley. I liked her right away and admired her for living alone in a loft in Soho, which she had redone herself with a great deal of invention and taste. I also admired her talent in art and the fact that she had a focus to her life—that she was working toward a specific goal. I envied the fact that she was doing all these things while still quite young. Linda and I enjoyed each other's company very much and we spent a lot of time talking and getting to know each other.

A very revealing beginning occurred when Linda brought out a cake box—the kind you'd see in a bakery, which are purchased flat but make up very quickly into a box and are tied with string. Leaving the box flat she asked me to draw on the outside with crayons a picture of my outside and on the inside a picture of what I looked like on the inside. I guessed that she meant a symbolic picture and drew on the outside a picture of the window of our apartment as seen from the street and also a picture of the layout of our apartment with my husband sitting in the living room and the kids in their bedroom.

On the inside of the box I drew a series of events which had occurred in a dream I had had the previous night and which I did not understand. The dream began with my seeing a brilliantly colored balloon on a string, floating in the air in front of our apartment building. The balloon had a clown face with a nose that lit up. The inscription "7D" was painted on the nose and each time it lit up there was an accompanying ring like that of a telephone. I reached for the string and was transported to the dark entryway of a tenement where I talked over an intercom to the man in 7D. A formless yet sinister man brushed by me going very fast. I told the man on the intercom that I was not willing to walk up the seven flights and was quickly transported to a pleasant tree-lined street where I took the arm of a gentle-faced policeman and we strolled along in the twilight, nodding at passers-by.

When I was finished I was completely surprised at what I had done. It was my first revelation to myself of "my secret life," of how much of myself I was keeping inside—my excitement and fascination with life, so much of me that is dark and frightening and even my distaste with being average, respectable and dull, which is in conflict with a fear of being shunned for being too emotional, excitable, wild, "loose."

When Linda and I had discussed the cakebox I began to see what art therapy was about, for it was not how or even what I drew that was important, but what my drawings meant to me and the story that I told about them and the story they told about me that was of major concern. As I said in the beginning of this paper, I've always wondered why I did certain things and I've always thought that the answer to the whys was important. In Linda I had found a person who was also interested in the whys.

It was almost frightening how the cakebox was like a picture of my inner self. Even I could see it. Maybe the things I was hiding were really more visible than I had thought. Maybe this hiding had something to do with my restlessness. Only now, over a year later, I am beginning to see how exhausting, futile and even damaging it is to try to hide that secret life from myself and others. My secret life—a life I see as exciting—(the balloon) attracts me greatly. But very soon I feel I'm getting in too deeply—I'm too committed (the dark hallway and the sinister man). I balk when I realize that the life I thought I wanted is too difficult or frightening (telling the man in 7D that I was not willing to walk up the seven flights) and I run back toward respectability (the policeman and the respectable walk along the street). That's the way I now see the dream. Certain questions presented themselves as a result of my view into my secret life: "Why must that life be secret? How can I bring that life into the open? Can that life be respectable in itself? What can I do about the pressures that forced that life into secret?"

At the end of every session Linda would bring out a piece of paper and crayons and I would make a mandala. The most interesting things about the mandalas to me were: what I could say about myself using this form of drawing; what things were more obvious to Linda because of her training; the progression over the weeks from helplessness and frustrated ideas to more positive ones being portrayed. I still enjoy making mandalas. Even though I can't really interpret them fully without help, I feel better just having done something about a feeling I have had.

We did some tentative work in making pots but they were not really what I wanted to do. I think I would have really enjoyed working on potter's wheel and then glazing pots, but these were all we could do without a lot of equipment.

Once when we were "playing" with the clay Linda asked me to portray my wonderful feeling of growth in some figure. I made a sculpture of a wave. I still love the symbolism of this. It is beautiful to feel like a wave—growing and growing and becoming bigger and more powerful and more exciting and frothier and curling over, about to become. Expectancy! It was wonderful to be able to show what I was feeling—to touch and form its perfect symbol—the wave.

The culmination of all our activities was the head of my father that I sculpted (with a great deal of help from Linda) and then cast in larger-than-life white plaster. This work required a great deal of time beyond our usual sessions and Linda gave freely of her time for many extra hours.

I decided on the head because I really had no desire to do anything else. Of all the visual art forms, sculpture seems to me to be the most impressive and interesting. I chose my father for many reasons which are still unclear to me but I have discovered many reasons in the process of making the sculpture and afterward. My reason at the time was the "you can have many husbands but only one father." What this says about my mother, sister and children and self, I don't know. But I do know that my father loomed large in my life and I just knew that it was only he that I wanted to sculpt.

It was this fact that began to take over in our sculpting sessions. As the head began to take shape out of the clay, I began to talk to it as if it really were my father. As Linda and I worked, molding and shaping and touching, we began to feel the presence of my father in the room.

I had never talked much to my father, never touched him, and here I was forming his features and hair, shaping and smoothing. It was a very sensual experience and a beautiful one. These sessions were long and exhausting and Linda and I would finish late at night, covered with clay or plaster, but having had a wonderful experience.

I would recall experiences from my childhood suggested by my father's presence and talk about my feelings about them. This would often lead Linda into a reminiscence which would produce new insights for her into her relationship with her father. It was almost as if we created a father who in turn taught us about ourselves. We used this father to reflect and absorb our feelings—pleasant and unpleasant— and we were able to express these feelings to our father openly and honestly, and, being the silent ball of clay that he was, he never disapproved or blushed or fought back.

But more wonderful than this was that I began to find that whenever I encountered my real father—the father of my youth who was so huge, and frightening and angry and embarrassed and withdrawn—I began to be more at ease about expressing my real feelings to him and found, much to my wonder, that so many of those qualities of aloofness and distance which I had ascribed to my father were the product of my never having communicated with him at all. When my feelings did not have the expected effect on my father—the anger or withdrawal I had anticipated—I was surprised to find him more real and less a huge and frightening figure.

My therapy with Linda began to taper off when my husband and I bought a house in Westchester. The head had not been completed and so I saw Linda a few more times to finish the actual work on the sculpture but it was too difficult and expensive for me to travel back and forth to the city.

I can't say that art therapy changed my life, but through a combination of events, my life is different and I know that everything I learn about myself and about life and my relationships with others helps to open doors for change. I have discovered within the past year that I want to devote myself to a career in singing. I have always loved to sing and always wanted to be a singer and always thought that it was too late or that I didn't have enough talent or that I wasn't beautiful enough. But encouraged by my analyst and Linda to seek my creativity and by friends to take some lessons, I have begun to really work on singing—to devote my time and energies to it.

The drive of that commitment seems to lead the rest of my life along—to strengthen me. Certain decisions which were difficult to face before making my commitment to singing are beginning to almost decide themselves as my life takes on a focus. As I pay attention to my creativity, as I allow it to take precedence in my life, it begins to bring my life together. I am still wondering and searching but now with some direction and much more certainty of finding something worth searching for.

A FREUDIAN PERSPECTIVE

Linda describes a woman down on herself, unsure of what she wants, and disconnected in her relationship with her husband. She feels unattractive, vaguely disoriented and frustrated in her life position. She approaches her art therapy relationship with an anxious hunger, searching to make contact but unable to really relate to the therapist except on a superficial, chatty level. At first, the art therapist, equally unsure of herself, allows the chatter to go on. Food is used as both a safe avoidance and perhaps a means of making safe contact for both patient and therapist. Gradually the two move towards more authentic engagement.

The patient shares some of her intimate sexual life. The art therapist feels uncomfortable. The patient expresses envy of Linda's lifestyle. Linda gives little interpretation but respectfully listens and waits. The dance soon takes on a more intense rhythm. The patient unconsciously depreciates herself and attempts to gain sympathy and support from the therapist. Fortunately, Linda gives neither. An old therapeutic axiom is employed: Do not respond to masochistic defenses with sympathy or pity. The patient's internalized criticizing mother, who attempts to set up others to feel superior to the patient and belittle her self-assertive moves in life, needs confrontation rather than appeasement. The art therapist is aware of these feelings and does not respond to the bait; in fact, she offers little or no interpretation. She does, however, share some of her own thoughts and confusions, and lets the relationship go forward. Deanna shares an initial dream. She draws the father figure—he is the clown, the amorphous image without a body, only a small appendage. Communication does not take place except by telephone. Another aspect of the father is the dark man who brushes past without speaking. There is also, however, a wish for a protective man who will help her cope with her wishes and dreams that are part of night. Is it possible to have a real and close relationship with a man that does not end up in a meaningless sexual encounter? Thus, a wish to communicate is given to the therapist as to some of her possible goals in treatment. Can Deanna bring together the various pieces of her life? Can the amorphous shadowy figure of the man in the hall come together with the protective policeman, the cartoon hand and the bodiless voice?

Essentially the patient gives a message to the art therapist: "Help me discover my real father—the good and bad father—the human father; give me the courage to touch and discover the male in my life." The therapist and patient begin a journey to discover lost parts of themselves. A frenzy of libidinal energy soon becomes released. The art therapist sets the stage for the patient to start identifying with a deep primitive part of herself. She calls forth from the patient an identification with the power of the ocean, the energy inside her, the deep maternal root of her past that is inextricably woven into her sense of self. Then the art therapist furthers the union by identifying with the rejected child-self. She speaks for this part of the patient and makes her come alive, supporting Deanna's need to be heard. Again there is a release of energy along with the pain of recognition. The patient looks at part of herself through role-playing while the therapist takes one more step in leading Deanna towards reorganization through the externalization of the rejecting mother. Together art therapist and patient take joy in her products, her creation. The implied communication by the art therapist states. "I like what you produce. I like what you give me. It is not feces but something beautiful." She molds and creates round and sensuous representations of parts of herself. The therapist supports the patient, helping her to accept the lost female self.

The mandala further reinforces the newly found power of becoming more centered and connected to her inner resources. The maternal introject seems unable to combat this new power within the patient. Indeed, she internalizes a new concept of herself mainly through encouragement and self-acceptance from the art therapist. Eventually creative energy takes form through the sculpture. Both the art therapist and patient dare to discover, touch and mold a new image of a male. He is touchable, malleable and communicative. Both share in the joy of creation. Both support each other's need for a father. Through clay a developmental experience is reconstructed, relived and realized. The female figure is not critical but supportive in the girl's wish to be close to the father figure, if only symbolically through the creation of a male.

The art therapist has some misgivings and starts to attack herself through her own dream. She is frightened of this newly found power within herself. A friend, sister and a grandmother are there within the group and somehow seem very much connected to making an accusation—"You are a bad therapist"—for daring to take on this power and authority. Of note, within Linda's dream there is no father figure.

Perhaps there is some underlying feeling of self-criticism. For Linda, in fact, takes over the father role within the therapeutic relationship. Yet, the therapist does not deny her power for long. The art therapy relationship continues with intensity illustrating the very complex interrelationship between self-development and creative development. Linda's case illustrates that there is no dichotomy between product and self-development. Both appear to go hand in hand. The relationship appears to create energy. The self is connected and the product becomes the manifestation of a new freeing and mastery of forces within and without the patient.

What seems evident are some of the more salient artifacts of an art therapy relationship. For one, it is a mutual journey for therapist and patient wherein both explore and perhaps share forbidden and lost parts of themselves. The creative act, with all its attending release of energy, becomes a focal point for new internalizations and a basis to affirm a new self through the act of creation (6, 7).

A JUNGIAN PERSPECTIVE

The Jungian viewpoint of the therapeutic dialogue between Linda and her patient, Deanna, differs in no substantial psychodynamic way from the expert and lucid critique by Dr. Robbins. However, a few differing emphases might illustrate the Jungian philosophy.

"Archetype" ("dominants," "primordial image," "imago") is the universal thought-form held to be common to many epochs and peoples. Jung subdivides the masculine principle into the basic archetypes of *father, son, brother, "puer eternus," hero, soldier* and *wise man*. Roughly comparable archetypes would be *mother, daughter, sister, "puella eterna," amazon* and *wise woman* (8). D. would seem a *"puella eterna,"* whose dominant archetype is the *great father*. Since her early development allowed her only an incomplete sense of *eros* or relatedness, she acted out relatedness in an immature, compulsively sexual way. The *puella* leads a life full of emotional wanderings and tentative attachments, with great difficulty in permanent commitment. Her animus (inner masculine principle) projects to the *hero*. Negatively, he constellates unrelatedness, aggression, destructiveness. Positively, a hero rescues a girl from the *father* and makes a woman of a maiden. Positively, the *puella* is concerned with and arouses the subjective individual aspect of herself and others (cf. her deepening relationship to R. and her increasing commitment to the art therapy process). Of note are the archetypal stages in Deanna's clay bust of "Dad": first, the *"puer,"* then the *hero*, then the *older man* (Spencer Tracy)—considered as R. for two sessions—and, finally, the *father*.

Jung chronicles the mystical royal marriage and the "coniunctio" in ancient culture, myth and alchemy, corresponding to the central significance of the transference in both psychotherapy and normal human relationships. "Dad's" emotional tie to D. seems clear; he responds by cutting off all feelings from a subject "too explosive to handle." D. responds by "feeling closer to Mom than to Dad," and choosing a husband in the father-image. Jung states: "Whenever the drive for wholeness appears, it begins by disguising itself under the symbolism of incest" (9). For unless he seeks it in himself, a man's nearest feminine counterpart is to be found in his mother, sister or daughter; a woman's in her father, brother or son.

The "decline" of Linda during D.'s four months of gratifying improvement is commonplace in the transference/countertransference dynamic of a therapeutic encounter, and perhaps constellates the archetype of the *wounded healer.* The patient brings her woundedness to the contract and the therapist her healing powers. With "mutual transformation," frequently the patient begins to experience *her* inner healing powers as the therapist does *her* woundedness. Clearly, D. helped Linda tap into her own troubled relationship with her father.

Jung pointed out that for *extroverted* types, psychic energy flows outward *to* objects, whereas for the *introverted,* energy flows inward *from* objects. That D. is clearly an extrovert and R. an introvert *could* be a plus for their marriage. When this basic attitudinal difference can be understood and assimilated, it can become a helpful complementarity (making for "good wrestling partners") rather than a baffling irritation.

The "typology" of Jung predicates four basic psychological functions: thinking, feeling, sensing, and intuiting. These are present in all of us to varying degrees, usually one being more highly differentiated ("superior"), and its polar opposite less consciously defined ("inferior"). The two others are "auxiliaries." Linda is probably an introverted sensation type with feeling as her second function (personal communication). Her intuition, as inferior function, is partly unconscious, but seemingly and luckily serviceable (her "push" and "risky ploy").

Unlike Freud, Jung looked at dream material as statements from the unconscious which either (1) compensate or complement a consciously-known position, or (2) restate for emphasis a factor not clearly understood. In this sense, they are often diagnostic or prognostic (as well as therapeutic), but we never accept an interpretation which is nothing but "confirmation" or "wish-fulfillment." The associations of the patient to any dream, therefore, are crucial. Often the *initial dream* brought to the therapist summarizes the task that life demands of the dreamer. I believe this may be the case with D.'s initial dream.

Unlike Dr. Robbins, I was fortunate in being familiar with Deanna's associations. The setting of the dream was her actual apartment in New York City. The dark stairwell was in a tenement across the street from her apartment. There are no special associations to Bozo the Clown, but red is the color of vivid feeling and affect. D.'s reaching for the balloon and following the "telephone" to the walk-up tenement building were felt by her as a strong attraction and pull; she was "being led" to a dark and dingy place. Although she had no personal associations to the apartment number 7D, she states that a "walk-up" apartment building in New York City is limited by law to six stories so that anything higher would be condemned. Her talk on the intercom is to a known man who asks her to enter a sexual relationship on a blithe, happy level, which she is not able to do. To this point the dream is in color. When the strange sinister man rushes in from outside, seeming to "fill the hallway with his presence," the dream switches to black-and-white, and D. shrinks against the wall in the darkness. The final scene (color again) shifts to the country—*not* New York City—and the friendly policeman is helpful and protective, like her husband. She feels respectable and "part of the community"; people in the street nod pleasantly to her and she to them.

An interpretation: D. is fascinated by excitement in general and by the "adrenalin" of New York City in particular. Following this beckoning path leads her into dubious and risky relationships in a "condemned" place. When up against the wall, D. *does* reach out for acceptance and responsibility. This D.'s husband constellates for her; part of her feels relaxed and at home in the country of friendly folk, while part of her experiences the going back from New York City to the protective country as a loss. D.'s task is to reconcile the two feeling parts of herself. The sinister intruder, frightening as he is, could be the bridge.

This interpretation or rephrasing of her associations won D.'s vigorous assent. It is worth noting that frequently the frightening intruder, far from being negative, constellates a very positive dream symbol, carrying something of great value. The animus often appears in dreams as multiple figures. (D. herself comments that Bozo the Clown, the man on the intercom, the Sinister Man and the friendly policeman were all male.) The sinister man from whom she currently shrinks in fear may ultimately be a reconciling symbol between the positive aspects of the exciting, vivid, forceful animus of the urban *hero*, on the one hand, and the warm, supportive and respectable animus of the small-town *wise man/father* on the other.

Linda's dream sounds like a warning dream: "To the extent that you allow the dialogue to become a group session, with the intrusive presence of your inner family figures, you *will* be dishing up an intoxicating brew of your own projections. STAY WITH THE DANCE!"

The therapeutic dialogue between patient and therapist can indeed, then, be transcendent and healing in and of itself, and for each. A final word on mandala symbolism: "D. told Linda to use her own medicine, and it worked." Jung adduces considerable data to show that whatever metaphysical or religious significance the mandala symbols have in many epochs and cultures, psychologically they all seem to express an attitude *to* or *from* the psychic center of the personality. That the circle can go either way is attested by the fact that the pictorial production of a mandala by an individual can either *arise from* contact with one's center, or *help reach* contact with one's center.

References

1. Stein, R. "The Incest Wound." *Spring—An Annual of Archetypal Psychology and Jungian Thought*, 133–142, 1973.
2. Castillejo, I. C. *Knowing Woman*. New York: Harper and Row, 1973.
3. MacNeill R. and MacNeill, G. *Open Marriage*. New York: The Avon Press, 1971.
4. See Chapter 17, Techniques, Function: Integration, Focus: Individual #14.
5. Jung, C. G. *Mandala Symbolism*. Princeton: Bollingen Foundation, 1959.
6. Freud, S. A *General Introduction to Psychoanalysis*. New York: Doubleday, 1943.
7. Freud, S. *The Collected Papers of Sigmund Freud*. London: Hogarth Press, 1953.
8. Jung, C. G. *The Portable Jung*. Ed. J. Campbell. Translated R. F. C. Hull. New York: The Viking Press, 1971.
9. Jung, C. G. *The Practice of Psychotherapy*. Translator R. F. C. Hull. Princeton: Princeton University Press, 1954, p. 263.

10. Play, Art and Photography in a Therapeutic Nursery School

Ellen Nelson-Gee

INTRODUCTION

I know a little what it's like to be a withdrawn child with Ellen as therapist—we once acted these roles out together and I vividly remember her comforting and unthreatening presence. Strangely, but not surprisingly, it was as easy for Ellen to become the child as it was for her to be the nurturing adult. I was reminded of this experience as I read her fieldwork account. It is not easy to describe the feeling I get from Ellen's description of her relationship with this vulnerable little girl, except to recall the nonverbal image of tall long-legged Ellen squatting way down to Terry's eye-view and looking at the world as she sees it. That kind of view could probably take your breath away.

Ellen listens to Terry's message as she repeatedly acts out behavior which broadcasts overwhelming feelings of impotence in an inconsistent and manipulative world. Ellen offers not only strength and non-mystifying communication, but also a way for Terry to play out what has been done to her and what she would like to do back to the sources of her paralyzing frustration. The extent of that frustration's effect is painfully illustrated in Terry's rigid board-like physical motion and contact and in her chronic constipation. The temperature-taking, the annihilation of their Polaroid photographs, the bandaids she places on her paintings—all are signs of serious needs which Ellen encourages to emerge through the safety of play.

Ellen skillfully handles some pretty sophisticated dilemmas. She subtly blends attention and love with non-reinforcement of attention-

The following five chapters were originally part of an unpublished thesis, *Dialogues in the Art Therapy Encounter*, edited by Heidi Sparkes and Arthur Robbins. The introductions are by Heidi Sparkes and the commentaries are by Arthur Robbins.

getting behavior. An example which Ellen herself points out is her turning Terry's interest towards more attractive activities rather than directing attention towards her "falling." Ellen patiently communicates physical receptivity but not aggression or intrusion so that Terry can begin to approach her—first through touch-and-go tactics, then through more direct physical contact and expressiveness. Ellen also combines firm treatment and guidance with her own vulnerability in play to give Terry an essential sense of self and power. The awareness and definition of these dynamics in Terry's behavior alone are an important learning process. To handle any one of these elements would have been a sufficient contribution. Ellen's ability to deal creatively and effectively with a number of problems exhibited by this complicated little girl makes this paper a classic one.

THE CASE—TERRY

The following paper is about a five-year-old girl who is one of six children in a therapeutic nursery class. I see her both privately and in her classroom, two days a week.

Terry is a lovely girl. She is five years old, has deep speckled grey-blue eyes, and, when she smiles, dimples. I met her in the fall of 1972. She came to the school late. The five boys in the therapeutic nursery class had been together a few weeks already. She became to them, alternately, a doll to fight over and share things with and a punching bag. This is how I first saw her. Her clothes were from an expensive store, and I am certain she was offered a well-balanced diet plus vitamins; yet she looked neglected, she was unhealthy, thin with pale skin. She had an habitual cold and runny nose, and she was severely constipated. She often sat on the toilet for long periods of time with no results. She complained, "My back hurts," and pointed to her buttocks. I first took her and a little boy, J., out of the room together for individual therapy; sucking her thumb, she would lie sometimes for forty minutes on the floor of the room we used.

At that time I was into what I now call my "togetherness" period. Whatever I was doing with J., I wanted Terry to participate in, and vice versa. Whereas both children may be, on paper, "minimally brain-damaged" and "emotionally disturbed," their behavior was as nearly opposite as I could have imagined. J. literally bounded from wall to wall; he tried to jump out the window and run into the street. Terry moved like a snail; she sniffled, whined and complained constantly about anything she was asked to do: "I can't." She "couldn't" open the door to her cubby, "couldn't" button her coat. This condition I call her "helplessness."

Once in a while, however, when J. was yelling in the hall or kicking a door, Terry would imitate what he was doing. He knew from experience that he could set her off like this, and he would start to yell and look at her out of the corner of his eye. Then she would look at him, smile and start doing just what he was doing. This was really frustrating for me. Yet how ironic: Here they were doing something

I would like especially to thank Pierre Boenig for being an excellent supervisor and a good friend to me. There were times when, but for his gentle and patient encouragement, I may have given up doing the work I was trying to do.

105

together . . . but not together-with-me. At those times I would try to assure Terry that she was indeed a different person from J. and did not have to do what he did. This may certainly have confused her; not ten minutes before, I had been encouraging her to do what J. and I were doing.

Perhaps what struck me the most about Terry when I first knew her was her resistance to being touched. If I took her hand, she would yell, "No!" and pull away. A hug made her body rigid and her face terrified. Connected with this, I feel, was her real concern over getting a spot of water or paint on her clothes. In the beginning she would just cry. Later she learned to say, "I want another shirt. I want another jeans." (Her mother kept a supply in her cubby.) It was as though contact with people's arms and faces, with paint or anything "mutti," as she says, would permit something to be taken away from Terry, would deplete her intactness. By staying rigid and touching nothing, she perhaps feels she cannot be hurt. Terry is extremely disconnected from her body which, in being a shell protecting the Terry inside it, is not a body allowed to defecate and be hugged and hug back and get dirty once in a while and be strong enough to perform what is required of it by the person inside.

Finally, I mention something which Terry brought to our first meetings along with her unhealthiness, "helplessness," imitativeness and resistance to being touched, but which I did not recognize until much later—her testing of me. J. was flagrant in his testing—hanging out the window or raising a block as if to throw it, all the time watching me as if to say, "Are you going to let me do this?" Terry's testing was much more subtle in the beginning, but I feel now that she, too, was asking for limits to be put on just that behavior which she brought into the classroom. I feel she was and is asking, "Are you going to let me get away with pretending I'm weak, copying instead of creating, resisting close contact with people who care about me?" I hope that I can show with some examples of our work together that my answer to her question is "no."

I began to deal with Terry's "helplessness" almost right away. In the fall, when she was told to put on her coat or open her locker or button her coat, her response was, "I can't," spoken with a whine. Lately she has been saying, "Ow, ow, ow," as if she is in pain, in order to get attention or to indicate that she "can't" do something. When I first noticed this "helplessness," I tried to encourage her by saying, "I know you can do it, but if you need my help you can ask me:

'I need some help.' " With this exercise, which we do together whenever she becomes frustrated by what she "can't" do, I am trying to help her to be in touch with her needs and to be able to communicate those needs to others. An example of this behavior occurred as we were walking through the park: *T:* "Ow. My shoe." *D:** "Does your shoe hurt?" *T:* "No." *D:* "Then what are you trying to tell me?" *T:* "Tie my shoe." *D:* "OK. You want me to tie your shoe." (I tied it.)

This kind of helplessness is, I think, fostered in Terry by her parents and her nurse. I feel there are many things she is just not *allowed* to do for herself—simple things like buttoning her coat or picking up a pencil or tying her shoe. She expects these things to be done for her, and she does not know how to ask for them appropriately when they are not done for her. Even I, who *know* that Terry can do many things by herself and many more things with a little help, almost got "conned" into doing something for her because of the helpless quality she exudes. We were sitting side by side on a bench in the park. She picked up a crayon and started to draw in her notebook, then she dropped it. I made a slight motion in the direction of the crayon: My instinct was to pick it up for her as I would pick up something anyone dropped. I stopped myself; she was watching me. *D:* "Pick up the crayon." *T:* "No, you pick it up." (She smiled.) *D:* "It's your crayon, Terry. You dropped it. You pick it up." (She did.)

I believe that, in part, Terry's acting helpless is a dramatization of how helpless she, in fact, feels. Her parents are large and overpowering figures. I have seen both her parents ignore what she has said or, worse, contradict something she has said which is the truth. One morning before school I came out of the cafeteria with a styrofoam cup of coke in my hand. Terry and her father were waiting for the elevator to go up to the classroom. Terry said, "Daisy! Can I have some coke?" Her father responded in a somewhat condescending manner, "That's coffee, Terry." I was slightly embarrassed to be drinking a "kid's drink" at 9:00 A.M. instead of a "grown-up's" drink, but I said, "As a matter of fact it is coke. Have some." I squatted down to Terry's level and saw then what 6'4" of Daddy looks like to 42" of child. My feeling is that Terry has resigned herself to the idea that if Daddy or Mommy says it's coffee, who is she to argue. So instead of arguing with her parent, she becomes him or her. By this, I mean she imitates the authoritative tone and manner of speaking of

---

* The author is called "Daisy" by her patients.

a parent. One day, Terry and I went outside together. We played in the sandbox. This is what happened:

T: "You, Daisy." D: You want me to go into the sandbox Terry?" (I went in and picked up a stick and squatted down, and started to draw lines and circles in the sand.) T: "I need a pail and shovel!" D: "We don't have a pail and shovel today, Terry. I'm going to use this stick to make pictures." (Terry also picked up a stick and made deep holes in the sand.) T: "This is Jan and Donna [her teachers] and J. and W. and E. [classmates]." D: "Where's Terry?" (She started poking the stick at me. I averted my face.) D: "Terry, don't poke that stick so close to my face." (She smiled and giggled and shook the stick.) T: "A temperature. Shake the temperature." D: "Oh, you're taking a temperature. Do you feel sick?" T: "Yes." D: "Where do you feel sick?" T: "Put the cream on, Daisy." (Her voice was very deep at this point. It sounded like an imitation of an adult's voice.) T: "No, don't move. Hold still, everybody, hold still." D: "You're taking a lot of temperatures." T: "Hold still, everybody. I'm taking your temperature." (She stuck the stick in my nose.) T: "In your nose." (Then in my ear.) T: "In your ear. Now in your *mouth*!" (Stuck it in my mouth.) D: "You're putting the temperature in a lot of places, Terry. Where does it really go?" (She poked it at my back.) T: "In the backside. It smells. Put the cream on." D: "How does it smell?" (She poked it at my back.) T: "Hold still." (Terry spoke in a deep voice; I sat still.) T: "It won't go in." D: "That's because you're not *really* taking my temperature. We're pretending. You pull your pants down when we really take a temperature." (I made two buttocks and two leg shapes in the sand and made a hole between the buttocks. I stuck in a stick.) T: "Make a birthday cake." D: "Yes, it does look something like a birthday cake with a candle." (I made a small mound and put a stick in it. She drew in the sand and stuck a stick in it. I drew a circle and told her it was a cake. I made the buttocks and legs again. This time she stuck the "temperature" in. Then she went back to sticking it in my back.) T: "It *hurts*!" D: "What hurts?" T: "My backside. Hold still. You be Terry." D: "OK. I'll be Terry. Who are you?" (She did not answer.) D: "Are you the mommy?" T: "Now hold still." (Deep voice.) D: "It hurts, Mommy." (She held the stick at my back and waited. Then she took it away.) D: "It's time to go now, Terry. We're going back to the classroom." (As we walked, she held the stick and

touched it to my back, just as when she was "taking my temperature.") *T*: "Hold still, Daisy." *D*: "Sometimes it's time to hold still,
Terry, and sometimes it's time to move. Now it's time to move." (We
continued on into the classroom.)

It appears that when Terry spoke in her deep voice and ordered me
to "Hold still," she became the parent, teacher, nurse or even class-
mate who wields power over her. At the same time, as if more clearly
to define her role, she made me into Terry. Another example occurred
the following week as we were playing with dolls and a "temperature"
I had made out of a plastic straw:

D: "Look what I've brought. A doll. Let's play with the doll." *T*:
"No." (I put the doll down on the floor and took out a plastic straw.)
D: "I'm going to take the baby's temperature." (Terry became interested.) *T*: "I'll do it . . . like this." (She took off the doll's pants
and shirt.) *T*: "Now lie down . . . don't cry . . . pull your pants down
. . . get a blanket." (She got a little cover, took off the big blanket
I had placed over the doll and put that on a bigger doll.) *T*: "Now
hold still: don't cry. Everybody can't get hurt. One more and that's it!
One more and that's it, Daisy." (She used the same deep, serious voice,
she had the week before.) *D*: "It hurts, Mommy. It hurts." *T*: "Hold
still. Everybody gets hurt. Everybody can't get hurt. Now hold still;
don't cry. Just one more and *that's it!*" (I picked up the Mother
puppet and the "thermometer.") *D*: "Now hold still, please. I'm
going to take your temperature." (The Mother puppet takes the
temperature of the doll.) "Now let's take the Mommy's temperature."
T: "You do it." (I put the Mother puppet down on the floor and
Terry stuck the "thermometer" up her dress.) *T*: "Now hold still.
Don't cry. Everybody can't get hurt. Just one more and that's it." (She
held the "thermometer" in place for a few seconds then took it away.)
D: "Now, Terry, it's time to stop our playing and go back to the
classroom."

Other episodes have occurred wherein Terry has asserted power over
what is even more helpless than she. During one session, the day we
started taking photographs together with a Polaroid camera, she put
all of the photographs we had taken so far (pictures of herself and of
me) in the sand and buried them. Another time, in the classroom, I
was holding a large rubber band, and she cried, "Break it! Break it!"
The next week, as we walked through the park, I saw some dandelions
growing in the grass. *D*: "Look at the dandelions, Terry." (She de-

liberately stepped on as many as she could.) *D*: "Do you feel like stepping on all the dandelions. You want to hurt them, Terry?" (She did not answer me.)

What I feel as still another manifestation of her helplessness is Terry's frequent practice of "falling" down as we walk, or if I chase her as she tries to run from me. The first time I remember her falling down like that was the day that we went to the sandbox. It was the first time she had left the room with me alone and without J., the boy I took out with her for the first few months. She had been sick with a cold for a number of weeks. As we walked through the building to go outside, she said that she wanted to run. *D*: "We run outside. Inside we walk." (I tried to take her hand. Terry fell to the floor and smiled. Then she got up and started to run again.) *D*: "No. We don't run inside. Running is for outside." (Outside, I took her hand and she fell to the sidewalk.) *T*: "You walk, Daisy. I'll run." (I let go of her. She started to run, all the time looking back at me. I ran after her and she fell down again.) *D*: "Terry, you're playing a game with me. Come on. Let's go to the playground." (Diversion away from the "falling" seemed to make her "forget" it momentarily.)

As I see it, her falling down is a sort of "sitdown strike" which says: 1.) No, I won't do it the way you want me to; 2.) I know this annoys you because you're always in a hurry and this will slow you down; and 3.) this will get me the attention I need. Because I see this behavior as a testing and attention-getting device, I try to respond to her by giving *her* rather than *her behavior* the attention she is demanding. For example, in this last episode, I tried to divert her attention away from falling down and toward the playground I know she loves. I did not say, "What's the matter?" "Why are you falling down?" Instead I said, "Terry, you're playing a game with me. Come on let's go to the playground." When she will not be diverted, however, and when her physical safety is concerned, I cannot pretend to ignore her "falling" in the hope that it will stop. The following is such a session:

I went to pick up Terry, and I could hear her mother telling her to answer the door. *T*: "It's Daisy!" (She opened the door and I went inside for a few minutes.) *T*: "J.'s not here." (We had not been out together with J. for weeks.) *D*: "No, J.'s at home, just like Terry's at home now. And now it's time for us to go out to the playground." (When we got to the street and I asked her to hold my hand while we walked on the street, she took my finger until we had crossed the street. Then she said that she wanted to run.) *D*: "OK. Let's run together." (She fell down onto the sidewalk.) T: "No." D: "Come on, Terry, let's go to the playground." (She ran to a wall and leaned forward against it, looking just like a little boy urinating against the wall. Then she crouched down and began hopping like a frog. T: "I'm a frog." D: "Yes, I see. Terry's pretending to be a frog, but she is really a little girl. I think it must be fun to pretend you are a frog. But I like Terry as a girl." (She fell to the ground again and dragged herself along the pavement, on her belly, just to the edge of the street.) T: "I'm a lion." D: "You are *pretending* to be a lion. You *look* like a girl. Come on, stand up and be a girl as we cross the street." T: "No." D: "I'm going to pick you up then and carry you across the street." T: "No." D: "Well then, you stand up and walk across the street with me." T: "No." (I wanted to pay less attention to her behavior, but I knew that I had to stay close beside her in case she tried to crawl into the street. The stares of the passers-by were not doing either of us any good, I felt. So, for these reasons, I picked her up, and carried her across the street, and put her down near the wall of Central Park. She again threw herself onto the ground.) T: "I'm a lion." D: "Would you like to go see the lion in the zoo?" T: "Yes." D: "Let's go this way then." T: "No." D: "OK. Daisy's going to climb over the wall here." T: "I want to climb." D: "Good. Come with me." (I climbed over the wall. She got onto the bench near the wall.) T: "I can't." D: "Do you need help?" T: "Yes." D: "You know how to ask for help?" T: "Help me climb." (I helped her over the wall. She fell to the ground again. This time I was not afraid that she would hurt herself if I ignored her and walked on, so that is just what I did. Pretty soon she came running up behind me.)

Terry's resistance to being touched has been fairly consistent since I have known her. I have described her "falling down" when I tried to take her hand on the street. Not only does she fall to the ground to avoid being touched or forced to go anywhere, but when she lies on the ground, she is deadweight—she appears to have no spine, no bones, no energy. Her change from a giggling, energetic, mischievous little girl to a lump on the floor is frightening to see. The following session took place recently:

As we started for the park, Terry lay on the floor, giggling and looking up at me. D: "Come on, Terry, let's go to the park." T: (giggling) "I wanna run!" D: "OK. You can run outside. Running is for outside." T: "I wanna *run*!" (She grabbed for the heavy bulletin board, almost pulling it over on top of her.) D: "No, Terry! I *will not* let you do that. Give me your hand and we are going outside." *T*: "No hands." *D*: "OK. You can take my finger when we cross the street." (She ran off and grabbed some postcards out of the rack where a woman was selling them, threw them on the floor, and then threw herself on the floor. It looked to me as if she had no bones in her body; the minute I would reach for her to stop her from running or doing something destructive, she would collapse onto the floor. She is afraid of being touched, I feel. I took her onto my lap and sat on the floor.) *D*: "Terry, you are not ready to go outside with me. We are going to go back to the classroom and stay there until you are ready to go outside with me." *T*: "No." (She struggled and kicked.) *D*: "Then we'll wait here until you are ready to go outside." (Finally she became physically calmer. She wasn't struggling in my arms and she sat quietly. I stood up very slowly and extended my little finger slightly at my side and waited for her. She took hold of it and we walked slowly out of the door and across the street.) *D*: "When we get to the park, you can let go of my finger and you can run." *T*: "No running." *D*: "Then you can stay with me." (I sat on the top step of the stairs which go into the park. She sat down next to me. I took out her book into which we had started putting photographs the time before and showed it to her.)

Certainly when Terry collapses onto the floor or pavement, she is exercising what little power she has in order to control the situation she is in. I take the lead from her; in our sessions I encourage her to make contact with me—that is, to be in control of the touching—rather than take the initiative myself. I have found that when I am calm and sitting still, she will come to me more readily than if I am moving fast, in which case she may run from me or fall down. If I hold my hand at my side and extend my little finger, she will quite often take hold of it; however, if I hold out my hand to take hers, she pulls her hand away from me and cries, "No!" In other words, I make myself physically receptive to her without being physically aggressive. I believe Terry craves warmth and affection like any other child, but is afraid of being swallowed up by overpowering mommies and daddies in the world. Thus, she must be allowed to seek warmth and bodily contact on her own terms. The following are examples of Terry meeting me in her own way:

Often in the gym or on the playground I would take Terry's hand, and we would run around and around yelling at the top of our lungs: "ONE TWO THREE FOUR FIVE SIX!!!" She always looked so alive when she was doing this, and I know I felt really good doing it with her. One day in the gym she asked me to run with her and I did, once around the gym. She said, "I want to run some more!" I was tired so I said, "OK. You run to the end of the gym and back to me and I'll wait for you." I sat on the floor with my legs spread open in front of me and my arms open wide to show her that *I* was waiting for *her*. She ran, in the stiff and unsteady way she runs, up to the wall and back towards me, laughing all the way. She ran straight to me, jumped into my arms, and knocked me over—both literally and figuratively. I was very surprised at getting so much physical contact from her. Then she said, "I wanna do it again." And she did, again and again and again, until other kids started imitating her, thus interfering with the pattern she had established. Her teachers were amazed as was I at her embracing me so apparently strongly. I say "apparently" because she was so stiff that holding her in my arms was like holding a piece of wood. And when I gave her a little tentative hug, instead of just containing her in my arms, she wriggled free. Again, she was in control of how much physical contact there was to be. I've seen her mother, when she comes to pick up Terry, literally swoop down from the sky and engulf Terry with an "Oooooh, Terrykins, give Mommy a greeeeat big hug!" At these times Terry cringes and goes stiff, just as she does when I try to hug her.

During morning playtime Terry came and sat next to me on the floor. I wanted to have some kind of contact with her whereby she could touch me actively and I could let her touch me passively: *D*: "Let's pretend that I'm a chair and you are going to sit in the chair." (I sat on the floor with my arms and legs stretched out. She sat stiffly on the floor between my outstretched legs.) *T*: "Let's be beds." (She lay down.) *D*: "I'm going to lie down on this bed [her]." (I put my head on her chest. She rubbed my hair softly.) *D*: "It's soft. It feels good. Shall I rub your hair?" *T*: "No!" (She put her string of beads in my pocket.) *T*: "Rub your back." (She rubbed my back.) *D*: "That feels good, Terry." (She reached up under my shirt.) *D*: "Rub on top of my shirt, Terry." (She tucked my shirt into my pants. A little boy, E., came over and sat very close to us. As Terry rubbed my back, I started to rub E.'s legs and to sing. Terry came and sat beside me. She was as close as she could get to me without touching me.) *T*: "I want to read." (She got the book about Horton, the elephant. We talked about each picture. She referred to Horton as she: She's doing this. She's doing that.)

I felt good about being so physically close with Terry. It was a little strange because we were in the classroom with the other children and teachers. Also, the psychiatrist who is the head of the therapeutic nursery program was in the room. But my feeling was that I just couldn't worry about what this one or that one was thinking. They would have to speak to me about it later if they thought I was doing something wrong. No one spoke to me. Later that same day when Terry and I were at the playground with the other children, an interesting thing happened which, I think, grew from the trust which Terry and I had built together that morning:

Terry got on the swing. I got on the swing next to hers. She got off her swing and came over and pushed me on my swing. *T*: "Don't come back." (I got off, walked off a bit, then got back on again. I thought at first that she really wanted *me* to go away; then I got the feeling that she wasn't talking to me but maybe to someone else to whom she wanted to say, "Don't come back." She pushed me again.) *T*: "Don't come back." *D*: "Leave me alone." *T*: "Leave me alone." *D*: "Go away." *T*: "Go away." *D*: "Put me where you want me to be." (She pushed me to the corner of the playground.)

I felt good because I had not taken her rejection personally. I felt that I could accept her telling me to go away without making her feel guilty for doing so. I feel that her exploration of me in the morning enabled her to push me away without fearing retaliation from me. In much the same way, Terry had explored and trusted me when we had the session in the sandbox and she was putting the "temperature" in my ear, nose and mouth. Finally, during a recent session, Terry showed me where she is in relation to touching me and where she wants me to be in relation to touching her:

I sat on a bench in the park. She started a ritual of running away from me to the far end of the bench, stepping up on it and walking over to me, stepping on my lap and continuing to the end of the bench, then running to the far end of the bench again and repeating the whole thing. *D*: "Terry, I don't like to be stepped on. It hurts. Will you step over me?" (This time she came to me and sort of fell across me and dragged herself over my lap to the end of the bench. I noticed that she was touching as much of me as she could—my face, my hair, my breasts, my lap, my legs. She repeated this about six or seven more times. Each time she climbed onto the bench closer to where I was sitting and hung onto me more as she crawled over me. I sat very still and made no attempt to hold her or contain her, except when it was necessary to keep her from falling from my lap onto the ground. She was almost deadweight as she crawled. She appeared to have almost no autonomy or control of herself. It felt as if she craved my body contact, but did not know how to get it. As she went by me again and again, I would greet her and tell her it was good to see her again. Then she started to step on me again as she went past me, non-verbally saying to me: "Are you still there? Do you care? Are you going to stop me?") D: "Terry, I don't like to be stepped on." (I was implying that Terry had the right to feel the same way.) D: "I like it when you touch me, but not when you hurt me. You can step over me and still touch me very gently." (She started to step over me a few more times.) D: "It's time to go, Terry." T: "No! I wanna run." D: "Go ahead. Run that way." (I pointed away from the street.) T: "I wanna run that way." (She pointed towards the street.) D: "Terry, run that way [away] and I'll go with you." (She started to run in the direction I had indicated and I ran after her. We both stopped at the bench with the notebooks and photographs and crayons spread out on it.) D: "Let's pick up our things and go inside." T: "No. I wanna run." D: "No, Terry. It's time to go back to the classroom and the other kids." (She walked a bit then said, "Carry me," and collapsed onto the ground, which was quite wet from rain.) D: "OK, Terry, I'll carry you across the street and then you can walk by yourself back to the classroom." (I tried to pick her up. She was deadweight—no spring to her. Finally I lifted her, carried her across the street, and put her down on the opposite side of the street. I extended my hand for her to hold. She took hold of my little finger and held it very tightly. We walked back to the classroom without incident.)

Only very recently have I given myself permission to reach out for Terry and hold her in my arms or in my lap when I feel she needs this physical limitation of her behavior. I hold her when she is acting out to the extent where, I feel, she is frightened by what she is doing and is possibly in danger of hurting herself or someone else. For instance, one time she was running around trying to pull things off of shelves and walls. I took her in my arms, held her in my lap, and talked softly to her, telling her we would wait until she was ready to go outside. As little as she appears to like being touched, I know that my holding her firmly helped her to organize herself. After sitting in my lap for a few minutes, she was able to get up and take my finger and go with me to the park.

I have mentioned that I feel Terry's apparent fear of getting messy is connected with her fear of being touched. I have tried gently to encourage her to put her fingers into "gooey" stuff which is not dirty, e.g., soap suds. The following is an example of such therapeutic play: We had a "tea-party" in the classroom. Afterwards, in the hopes of getting her to get her hands into something which was "gooey" and clean, I asked her if she wanted to wash the dishes. T: "No." D: "OK. You fixed lunch; I'll wash up." (I took the dishes to the sink and ran it full of sudsy water and dumped the dishes in. Terry came over and took over the washing operation.) T: "Wash the baby's hair." D: "You want to wash the baby's hair, too. OK. Finish washing the dishes first." (She ignored this and went to get the baby doll. She put the baby into the water with the dishes. She washed the baby's hair for about five or ten minutes. She kept sudsing and sudsing his hair and rinsing and sudsing. She appeared really to be enjoying herself.)

Two days later Terry set up a tea-party by herself and invited me to come. T: "Daisy, come to a tea-party." (She had set up plates, cups, a pot of "tea," plastic fruit on a plate.) D: "I've brought some crackers to eat." (She put a piece of fruit on each of our plates. We "ate" and drank for a short time, then Terry said, "Let's wash the dishes," just as I had said two days before. We took the dishes to the sink, and she filled the sink with sudsy water and dumped in the dishes. The baby followed close behind. She repeated the cycle of washing, scrubbing and rinsing; washing, scrubbing and rinsing, just as she had before.)

Terry's disconnection from her own body as well as from the bodies of others is apparent in her drawings made in the following session: Terry was at the chalk board. She started drawing with a sponge, then with the chalk. T: "This is a circle (face). This is the eyes . . . nose . . . mouth . . . body . . . legs . . . feet . . . ears . . . hair . . . the chin . . . the chin . . . the chin . . ." (Each "chin" she added was a line coming out of the head.) T: "It's a sun!" (Indeed it looked like a sun.) T: "I want another shirt." (She had gotten a little water on her shirt. The teacher came over and said she could change her shirt when she was finished at the board. T: "I'm finished." D: "Terry, let's have a tea-party." T: "No." (She set one up later that afternoon.) D: "Would you like to play with blocks?" T: "No." D: "Let's draw on paper." T: "No." (I took out paper and crayons, anyway, and sat down at the table. She came over and started to draw rapidly, making about ten drawings in about twenty minutes.) T: "Here's the circle . . . the eyes . . . the nose . . . an ear . . . another ear . . ." (and on, just as on the chalk board). Her drawings are very bizarre, and they give a very clear picture of her extremely poor perception of her body (see Figure 10.1).

The first drawing was a picture of "Mommy." A larger circle was the head; a smaller one was the "body." Two sticks coming out of the body she called "the legs." Two large empty eyes, a line for a nose, a small mouth and two circles for ears comprised the face. The many "chins" protruded in all directions from the face and even ran through the face as if to scratch the whole thing out. (I once saw Terry take a newspaper engagement picture of a young woman who looked not unlike her mother and smear the whole face with paint. She did the same thing to another photograph of a young woman on the same newspaper page, and another, and another. It was frightening to watch this fragile-looking little girl destroy these smiling, pretty— although posed and a little phony-looking—faces.) The second picture was "Daddy and Mommy." Their many "chins" made them look like pincushions. I asked her which was Daddy and which Mommy, but she did not make that clear to me. One of the figures was only a head. The other had the same sort of body she gave "Mommy" in the first picture. The next picture was of "Mommy" and "G.," her seven-year-old brother. She put a piece of tape on "Mommy's" face. The next was of "Daddy." His many "chins" looked distinctly like a beard. I asked Terry if she could show me her chin. She pointed to her chin. D: "Does Daddy have a beard?" T: "No." D: "Does Daddy's face feel rough sometimes?" T: "Yes." (Then she put a piece of tape on Daddy's face.) D: "Oh, what are you putting on Daddy's face?" T: "A band-aid." D: "Did Daddy hurt himself?" T: "Yes." D: "What did he do?" T: "He hurt himself." D: "Did he cut himself shaving?" T: "Yes." D: "And now you put a band-aid on it for him. Does it feel better now?" T: "Yes."

Terry continued to make drawings and add band-aids. One was of "Mrs. B.," her nurse. "Mrs. B." had a neck and a band-aid on her hair. D: "Who is that, Terry?" T: "Mrs. B." D: "What hurts on Mrs. B.?" T: "She cut her hair." (What a fantastic connection to make between needing a band-aid because her Daddy cut his chin and needing one because Mrs. B. cut her hair.) D: "How does Mrs. B. feel now?" T: "Good." (The next picture was of "Daisy." She put a band-aid over part of Daisy's mouth. I thought, "Oh boy, she wants to shut me up so I won't ask her any more questions!") D: "What hurts Daisy?" T: "Her pee-pee." D: "Then put a band-aid on Daisy's pee-pee." (She put a band-aid on the middle of my "body.") Terry had often com-

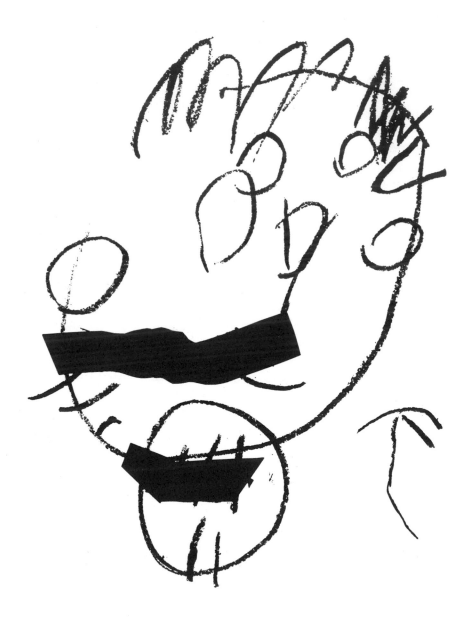

FIGURE 10.1: This drawing by five-year-old Terry could have been done by a child of three years. The primitive rendering of the head and the absence of a body suggest a poor body image. The eyes are vacant and sad. A band-aid has been placed over the mouth, perhaps as protection against invasion of food or the feared thermometer.

plained, "My pee-pee hurts." My feeling is that when she said that Daisy's "pee-pee" hurt, she saw no separation of herself from Daisy.

The next picture she drew was of the "Burger King" (Figure 10.2). She put tape over "Burger King's" mouth. *T*: "Take her temperature." *D*: "You want to take Burger King's temperature? Is she sick?" *T*: "No." *D*: "What hurts?" *T*: "Her pee-pee." (My feeling here is that Terry feels invaded by the thermometer when her temperature is being taken. Perhaps she put the tape over Burger King's mouth in order to prevent the intrusion into either her mouth or her anus.) *D*: "Terry, does your pee-pee hurt you?" *T*: "My pee-pee hurts." (At that point she saw a ruler lying on the table.) *T*: "Temperature!" (She picked it up and drew a straight line with it and put a small circle at one end of the line.) *D*: "That looks like a temperature, Terry." (Then suddenly she pushed the crayons and paper away and would not draw anymore. She started playing with some plastic blocks which are much more rigid, the compulsive-type of toy she usually plays with, as opposed to the relatively freer medium of crayons and blank paper.) Later that day when we were playing with the baby doll, she took some tape and put a "band-aid" on his penis. *D*: "Does the baby feel better now?" *T*: "Yes."

Later, I worked with photographs we took together to try to get Terry to look at and experience her body doing things: *D*: "I'm going to take a picture of Terry playing in the sand." (I took the picture and pulled it out of the camera.) *D*: "Look, Terry, what do you see?" *T*: "Terry." *D*: "Yes, I see Terry's feet, Terry's knees, Terry's smile, Terry's ribbon." *T*: "Terry's jeans, Terry's arms." *D*: "Terry's hair." *T*: "Terry's teeth. Terry's gum." *D*: "Yes, Terry is chewing gum. Now I'll take a picture of Terry chewing gum." (She started chewing in an exaggerated way. I took the picture and showed it to her.) *D*: "What do you see?" *T*: "Terry's chewing gum." (She took all of the pictures I had taken of her, put them in the sand and covered them over with sand.)

The following occurred in another session. *T*: "I want a picture of Terry." *D*: "OK. I will take a picture of you." (She looked at the camera, and I took the picture and showed it to her.) *T*: "It's another Terry." *D*: "It's the *same* Terry. It's *another picture* of Terry." *T*: "I want a picture of Terry." *D*: "OK. I'll take *another picture* of Terry." (I did.) *T*: "It's another Terry." *D*: "It's the same Terry. It's another picture of the same Terry." *T*: "I want a picture of Terry looking at the pictures." *D*: "Let me take another picture of Terry looking at the

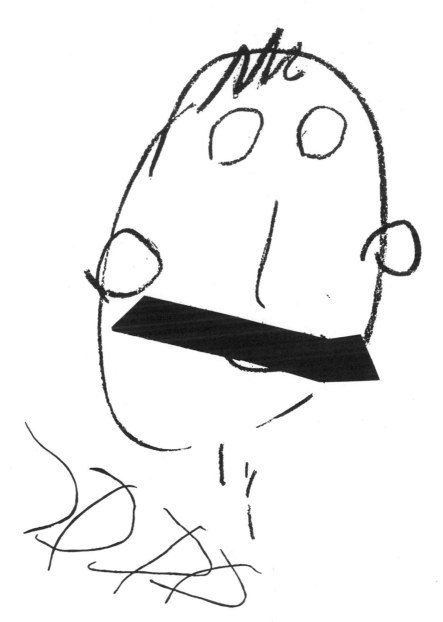

FIGURE 10.2: Terry said this picture was of "Burger King." She put tape over "Burger King's" mouth. *T*: "Take her temperature." *D*: "You want to take Burger King's temperature? Is she sick?" *T*: "No." *D*: "What hurts?" *T*: "Her pee-pee."

pictures." (I did.) D: "Who do you see?" T: "Terry looking at the pictures." D: "That's right. Terry is looking at the pictures."

Later I added a new dimension by using a mirror as well as photographs to help Terry see her body and what it does. We sat together, alone in the classroom. The other children were on the playground. T: "I want a picture of Terry." D: "OK. I'll take a picture of Terry." (She was smelling the photo emulsion on her finger at the time.) T: "It's mutti." D: "I'm taking a picture of Terry smelling her finger and saying, 'It's mutti.'" (She looked at the picture.) T: "I want a picture of Terry." D: "I'll take another picture of Terry smelling her finger." (She put her finger to her nose and said, "It's gooey." I took the picture and she looked at it.) T: "It's another Terry." D: "It's the same Terry. It's another *picture* of Terry." T: "I want a picture of Daisy." D: "You can take a picture of Daisy." (She held the camera and I helped her point it at me.) T: "It's another Daisy." D: "It's another *picture* of Daisy." T: "I want to take another picture." D: "There's no more film in the camera." (She ran to the window and looked out. D: "What do you see?" T: "P J. and there's J. on the playground." D: "Yes, you can see all the kids on the playground. Do you wish you were outside with them?" T: "No. I want to buy some more film." D: "We will buy more film for Thursday, but you can play with the camera without the film. Would you like to do that?" T: "Yes. Play with the camera." (She picked up the camera and looked through the viewer out the window.) D: "What do you see?"

I then brought over the pictures we had taken so far to review Terry's self-image. I held up the one I took of her smelling her finger. D: "See the picture. See Terry. What is Terry doing?" T: "It's mutti." D: "Yes, Terry is smelling her thumb and saying, 'It's mutti.' Can you do that like you are doing in the picture?" (I put my thumb to my nose. She put her thumb to her nose.) T: "It's gooey." D: "Yes, it was gooey. And look at this picture (of her chewing gum). What is Terry doing here?" T: "Gum!" D: "Yes, Terry is chewing gum. Can you see Terry's teeth?" (I touched the picture of her teeth.) D: "Can you touch your teeth?" (I opened my mouth wide and showed my teeth. She imitated me. I touched my teeth. She touched hers.) D: "Come, let's go to the mirror and bring our pictures with us." (I was surprised that she readily came with me. We sat together on a wooden box close to the mirror.) D: "Here is the picture of Terry smelling her thumb." (She looked at it.) D: "Now Terry can look at herself smelling her thumb. Put your thumb to your nose." (She did. She looked at herself intently. Then she got up and ran to get some animal crackers left over from lunch. She sat eating the crackers and looking at herself in the mirror.) *D*: "Now here is a picture of Terry chewing gum." (She looked at the picture.) *D*: "Now you can see Terry in the mirror. She is chewing." (She looked at herself and smiled.) *D*: "Now Terry is smiling. I can see her teeth." (I started to sing.) *D*: "Put your finger on your teeth, on your teeth." (I put my finger on my teeth; she imitated me).

Terry and I continued with this body-image song, touching all parts of our bodies. For once Terry seemed to have forgotten her physical defensiveness. Then she began to sing the song that we all sing at juice-time. *T*: "J.'s at the table, J.'s at the table, J.'s at the table having some juice." *D*: "Who else is here?" (She sang to two other children in the class.) *T*: "Daisy's at the table . . . no Daisy, Terry. Sing to Pat" (a student-teacher who had left). (I waited, expecting Terry to sing. She did not.) *D*: "You want me to sing to Pat?" *T*: "Yes." *D*: "Pat's at the table, Pat's at the table . . ." *T*: "Pat's not here." *D*: "Oh, Terry, you fooled me." (I now feel bad about my response. I feel I should have pursued the subject of Pat's absence. After this song, it was time to go.) *D*: "It's time to go now, Terry. Your Mommy's waiting." *T*: "No!" *D*: "Yes. Let's go see if we can find her."

I was not fully conscious of the extent to which Terry was and is testing me until I had been working with her for many months. In the very beginning, she spoke so little, and then only to imitate someone else. So when she started saying things like, "I want to run," and "I want to stay," and "Do this, Daisy," I was so pleased with her self-assertion that I failed to see that she was trying to discover how much she could manipulate me. I do not think there is anything wrong with allowing a child, especially one so damaged and powerless as Terry, to wield some power over an adult. I do feel, however, that it is important for the adult to be aware of the fact that she or he is being manipulated. A recent session was a turning point for me in the recognition of and connection with the game Terry was playing:

We were sitting in the park. We had just finished taking a roll of film, and she was sitting with her notebook and the photographs in her lap. She took all of the pictures out of the book, unrolled the tape which I had prepared for her to attach her pictures, put the tape in the book, and stuffed all of the pictures in the book. I took a pencil to make some quick notes and she took the pencil out of my hand.

T: "That's my pencil." (She smiled.) D: "You may use that pencil. I have another." (She started to scribble and draw in her notebook. I took out another pencil.) T: "That's Terry's pencil." D: "No. I am going to use this pencil. You have another pencil." (She scribbled in my notebook and looked up at me and smiled.) D: "Terry, you have your own notebook to write in." (She put a picture—the first photograph of her—in her notebook and traced around it. Then she scribbled on a few of the pictures she had taken of the fence in the park. She appeared to be more interested in the pencil, book, and tape than in the photographs.) T: "I want some more tape." D: "You have enough tape, Terry." (She drew some pictures in the book.) D: "Who is that you are drawing?" T: "It's Terry." (She wrote her name *backwards* and spelled it out loud.) D: "You wrote your name. Terry. And now it's time to go and find the other kids." T: "No." D: "What do you want to do?" T: "I wanna stay in the park." D: "It's time to go, Terry. Come with Daisy while she moves her car, and then we can find the other kids in the park."

It is probable that Terry would have kept asking for each of my pencils had I continued to give them to her. She drew on my notebook, then looked at me and smiled. She wanted a reaction from me—anger or merely a limit to her mischief? When I told Terry that it was time to go, she said, "No." I have the feeling that she said "no" more because she likes saying "no" than because she did not want to do what I had suggested. With the word "no" she has the power to direct or change events; the word "yes" suggests compliance with what someone else has determined will happen. Having begun to connect with Terry's attempted and sometimes achieved manipulation of me, I was able to observe what she was doing with a little more distance the following week:

D: "We're going out of the room now. We're going to play together now." (We left and went towards the elevator. I was carrying crayons and her notebook. I gave her her notebook to carry.) D: "We're going upstairs now." T: "I wanna stay here." (She sat down on the floor, opened up the book, and took the pictures out and spread them out on the floor. People kept walking past us and staring at us.) D: "Terry, we can stay here in the hall, but we'll have to move to this corner." T: "OK." (We went over to the corner and Terry said:) "I wanna go to the park." D: "OK. Get your coat and we'll go to the park." (I wanted to go to the park, too, so I did not really connect with her testing of me at this point. We got our coats and went down to the ground floor. She got out of the elevator and started to run through the halls. I dropped what I was carrying and went after her. She started to run off again. I held her in my lap.) *D*: "You're not ready to go to the park yet. We'll wait here until you are ready. Let's look at some of your pictures." (We spread the photographs out on the floor. She looked at them for a few minutes.) *T*: "I wanna run." (She giggled and looked at me.) *D*: "You can run when we get outside in the park." *T*: "I wanna run now." *D*: "Come with me and get your notebook I left in the hall." *T*: "No." *D*: "Do I have to carry you?" *T*: "Carry me."

I picked her up, carried her to the hall, picked up her notebook, and went back to the door. Terry continued to test me. *D*: "Are you ready to walk by yourself now?" *T*: "No!" *D*: "I'm going to put you down." (I put her down. We went out the door and she started to run up the sidewalk toward the street. *D*: "Terry, I'd like you to hold my hand when you're on the street." *T*: "No!" *D*: "OK. Then I'm going to stay very close to you." *T*: "No." (She ran and I stayed with her. She stopped and fell down to the sidewalk.) *T*: "No running, Daisy." *D*: "You want Terry to run, but not Daisy." *T*: "Carry me." *D*: "You want me to carry you. All right. I'll carry you across the street." (She was telling me what she needed; she wanted me to touch her.) *D*: "Now I'm going to put you down and we can go into the park." (She stopped at the benches.) *D*: "Let's stay here." (I put the notebook and photographs and crayons down on the bench.) *D*: "Here are pictures we took last time. And here is your book." *T*: "Take some pictures." *D*: "No. We're not going to take pictures today. We're going to look at the ones we have now." (She opened the notebook and started to draw in it with the crayons.)

It is clear to me now that in the beginning of the session I allowed Terry too many options. I went along with her every time she changed her mind: "All right, we'll stay here; OK, we'll go to the park." It was right after we began to visit the park that I realized she could, and probably would, keep thinking of new places she wanted to go or different things she wanted to do—as long as I never said "no." In one session, I decided that we would go to the park, no matter what diversions she engaged in *en route*. Eventually we did get to the park, and Terry was able to ask for help along the way by asking to be carried. We then had a beautiful session, which I have described, when she began climbing on me and running away and coming back and climbing on me again and running away again. I feel she needs to know that I care enough about her to say "no" to her self-destructive behavior and to *stay with* and *enforce* my "no." Her teacher, subsequent to this session, told me that she has seen Terry's mother deny Terry certain things and then give in as Terry began to cry. Terry must learn that she can trust me to be consistent in my demands so that she may learn to be consistent in her reactions to these demands. I feel also that in my being consistent I am giving her, in a sense, a picture of who I am and what she can expect from me. A natural result of her experiencing this will be, I hope, her experiencing who she is—first in relation to me, and then by herself.

COMMENTARY

Ellen's report offers an artistic and creative style in her soft engagement of this very disturbed and provocative child. I cannot separate what I know of Ellen in class from what I experience of her in the report. She is the sad clown, piercingly and poignantly carrying her message with a degree of lightness and love. As Heidi points out, she can be equally at home with both the adult and the child role. Often it is the case that a good child therapist has readily available the child-self within to be freed and expressed at the appropriate moment. Ellen utilizes her own child-self to make contact with Terry. She sensitively understands how easily this child can be invaded, intruded upon, or used.

Terry comes from a family where power is the medium of exchange. As a means of coping with a very overwhelming situation, Terry employs helplessness and submission as a powerful tool to manipulate and control her environment. Ellen is wise to this and treads the very delicate line of protecting her from her own self-destructiveness, while simultaneously giving her enough room to develop ways of coping other than passive helplessness.

Ellen attempts to avoid power fights with a child who is full of provocativeness and who challenges the therapist to play this overwhelming role. Ellen sidesteps, plays, charms, and lovingly offers tenderness and responsiveness as an alternative to willfullness. Through the medium of the sandbox, Terry plays out her deep fears of being intruded upon. Passive-submissive feelings are expressed by this girl and Ellen gives her latitude for control and mastery over very difficult and humiliating feelings. Indeed, the entire encounter is directed at giving her a sense of her own autonomy. She plays out the "no" and enjoys the delicious sense of control over Ellen. She uses the therapist as an instrument to admonish her parents. With each step that Terry takes toward separateness, her fears about separation and abandonment are stimulated. Thus the very complicated demand is made upon the therapist: Let me be free but show me you care. Ellen comes through this task with flying colors. She holds the child with care and tenderness rather than confinement and restriction.

Very basic issues are being attended to in this relationship. Ellen skillfully uses the tool of a mirror and camera to initiate a rebuilding of this girl's body-image. One has the sense that Terry feels as if her body were a disgusting thing. They take pictures of one another, mirror one another, explore each other's bodies, and perform many of the basic functions of a good mother-child relationship. Ellen essentially is attempting to give this child a more positive feeling about her libidinal self. Thus, as they touch various parts of one another, there is a beautiful feeling of tenderness and engagement. The child dares to confront the parental disgust that is lodged within her. Soon there are even signs in Terry of joy about her body rather than repulsion with it.

As Terry has been subject to a good deal of power and manipulation games, it is no surprise that she likewise exercises more than her share of sadism. This is a common pattern in disturbed children which occasionally causes difficulty on the part of the therapist. The therapists who are responsive to the deprivation and damage of their patients may find it difficult to also attend to the patient's need for power and reactive wishes to manipulate and torture others. Ellen soon discovers this in her patient and is able to limit her with care and tenderness. She soon understands also the importance of consistency.

Sexual identification issues become prominent as we observe the dialogue between Terry and Ellen. Terry has already begun to associate femaleness with subjugation and wishes to be the subjugator who has the power and control. Ellen starts to touch upon this area and will need to expand this issue as they become more intensely connected in therapy.

After reading this report, I feel a deep sense of pride and satisfaction in the work of this student. It is fortunate that her report does not lie buried in our files. The joy, tenderness, and creativeness of Ellen should be shared with other art therapists who have not had the pleasure of knowing her or her work.

11. Art Therapy in a School for Mentally Retarded Children

Joan Ellis

INTRODUCTION

The richness of Joan's interaction with her retarded children—her multiply-handicapped misfits—seems to be her inexhaustible capacity for emotional investment in these girls, as well as the empathic imagery with which she perceives them. The poignancy of this situation is the contrast of their warm growth-nurturing therapeutic environment and the less supportive outer-reality, that of working within an institution and with people who are less sensitive to the communication that is going on here.

The therapeutic environment which Joan has created and described is definitely an inviting one—I get the feeling of a soft, cornerless, pulsating room in which each child is unfolding at her own speed. It is obvious that Joan feels the benefits to be mutual and the feeding to be reciprocal; these children seem to be life-enriching for her. If not, it would be difficult to imagine her handling them so individually and so tenderly. Another image comes to mind—that of a skilled juggler who is enthusiastically managing a number of different feelings, goals, and responses . . . weaving them in and out of a unique and meaningful pattern, intuitively trusting her senses and skills. Joan sensitively deals with various complicated problems: using clay, paint, music, and dance to give sensory-training, self-mastery, and pleasure; picture slides, showers, and cosmetics for self-image and reward; behavior modification techniques for otherwise impossible control and coordination; and her own voice and body to express security and encouragement.

Much of what I have found to be most difficult in learning this art—staying open to overwhelming or unappealing feelings, demanding my rights from superiors or at least directly expressing dissatisfaction when nothing else could be done—Joan seems to take for granted. What she has most brought home to me, however, is almost too subtly exhibited here: From the careful and competent ordering of so much input, one might overlook the potential chaos of this situation. In actuality, Joan's maturity is most demonstrated by her facing this chaos—allowing it to flood her rather than prematurely closing or structuring her responses. Watching Joan openly hassle in supervision with each step of her development with each child and grapple with the unsympathetic setting at her placement, I became more aware of the need to feel and to share the frustration, anger, and boredom which can disconnect anyone from important sources of therapeutic response.

THE CASE—"MISS ELLIS' REJECTS"

Robin

So much has happened since the first report on "Miss Ellis' Rejects."* For one, Robin had been out of school for several weeks as one of the victims of an epidemic of lice and nits affecting the school. Frequent calls to her home by the nurse, describing treatment, were of no avail. The mother kept returning her to school, the nurse would check her hair, find the colony of nits increased, and take her home. The mother would send in notes saying, "I've washed her hair; she's clean; she's driving me crazy."

For hours the poor child would sit in the nurse's office looking totally lost. I would stop in to see her, tell her how much we missed her and that we would wait for her to come back. She always responded with "Joanie, I'm back," or "I belong to you, Joanie."

Robin was out for a total of 56 schools days. She returned at the end of January and seemed to be no further advanced than at the beginning of the school year. The only difference—and a very important one—was that she seemed to have a sense of being a part of the class and "belonging" to me. She constantly watched me for my responses and reactions. Though she felt a belonging—she came in, looked around, said hello to everyone—she nevertheless had a questioning look about her, possibly because there had been so much growth within the group while she was gone.

There are no specific routines in the morning now. The girls know what they want to do when they come in and don't need specific directions from me for the first period in the morning. Anna might take a brush and can of water and paint on the blackboard. Sharon will put a record on the player. Ellen might watch herself in the mirror or look at a picture book she brought in rather than exhibit her earlier autistic behavior by running around and around a table. Clara might take paper and crayons from the supply closet and draw. Theresa might also draw or engage in some other activity while wait-

---

* These preadolescent and adolescent girls are students who have been unable to function in regular special education classes. This is the second report of this art therapist with these students.

ing to go into another class where she will spend the morning doing academic work.

Robin, however, goes back to her peg board and randomly puts in the pegs. I expect that there won't be any visible growth for a while. But, nevertheless, I am upset at the lack of growth and went to yell at her sometimes. I think about the notes her mother sends. I remember the original information on Robin: how she is kept away from her uncle and aunt; how she strongly represses all of her emotions, particularly anger; how she smiles, her façade, trying to be the sweet child everyone will love.

I listen to the mumbled conversations she has with herself. I wish I could put a microphone to her mouth to find out the specifics of what she says—how she keeps herself from becoming lonely. Robin is the only one Robin has. Basically she relies upon herself, which is too great a responsibility for her. I finally realize how extremely closed-off she really is. We have come one step together, however, and she does feel a sense of belonging to me. But she has not reached a point where she can share her feelings—her anger. I wish she would throw a tantrum but I'm afraid to provoke her. Her whole life has been a series of provocations and punishments, large and small. The long separation from school this year has been very bad for her. If she had stayed, at this point she might have been able to develop a closer relationship to me and we would have moved from there. But now I see the same frightened, mask-like smiling, rigid, controlled child whose only positive sense of the world is her feeling of belonging here.

We turn out the lights, take off our shoes, put on "The Theme from Fantasia" record, and we begin to dance movements. Robin just stands there. Verbal encouragements to join us do no good. I take her arms in mine and she pulls back. I get her to lie on the floor next to me. She stays close until I begin to slowly move my body. Then she moves away. I show her how to lie on her back and bring her knees to her chest. All the while she mumbles to herself, constructing emotional security and perhaps barriers. I take both her legs and push them in and out, in and out in time to the music, simultaneously giving her a great deal of verbal praise. She can stand this only a minute, then moves away to put on her shoes, smiling as if to say, "Okay, now I hope you like me since I've done what you want me to do."

Anna

Anna momentarily tunes into the music and moves her body in
rhythm. She tunes out, her movements become erratic. She tunes in,
her movements become rhythmic. Her extremely hyperactive behavior
—her inability to focus on objects, persons, anything—has begun to
diminish. Through my setting up a daily situation for Anna which was
failure-free, she has begun to experience and develop a sense of herself.
I've tried to set up a program that offered her different opportunities
to experience success. She is allowed the freedom of movement, action,
interaction, reaction. At other times some minimal structure is imposed upon her.

Behavior modification techniques were first used to help Anna
develop controls. A task was set up which required her to sort different-colored beads. She worked up to sorting six colors. Behavior
modification has been very successful with Anna. We set up a cardboard "corral" on her desk which blocked off three sides of the room.
Anna is so severely perceptually-impaired and distractible that it was
necessary to give her this additional external control to assist her
initially before any controls could be developed within herself. We
began by sorting out two colors. As she began to experience complete
success through verbal praise and tangible positive reinforcement such
as food, we built her up to sorting three, four, five and six colors. Considering her past history, the amount of control Anna began to place
upon herself was incredible. She felt the success in finally being able
to accomplish a perceptual-motor task. I then devised a system to help
her string different-colored beads. She was given two colors of beads—
which were also differently shaped—in one large cup. In front of that
were two empty cups. In front of each cup was a color card corresponding to the color of each bead. In step #1, she was to sort out the
two color beads into their respective cups. During any sorting task, I
find it especially important to continually verbalize, "Pick up *one*
bead, *feel* the one bead." This helps to eliminate her tendency to grab
handfuls at a time. Then, in step # 2, she was asked to pick one bead
out of each cup and place it on its corresponding color card. She was
told to string the beads from the card, not from the cup. By starting
from the card on the left, she would place that bead on the string
and then move to the card on the right. For the first time in her life,
Anna was able to string alternate beads of two different colors.

The majority of the teachers in the school use the Frostig Program of Perceptual Development. I too have used it successfully with some children. Unfortunately there are many like Anna who are so severely impaired that they could not even focus on a pencil. The Frostig program was too great a threat to impose upon a child like Anna.

Painting has proved to be extremely successful in her visual-motor development. We began with a large sheet of paper, a large brush, and two bright but contrasting colors. Anna was first allowed to paint any way and anywhere on the paper she wanted to. After she began to show a feeling of freedom and confidence using these materials, a structure was again imposed upon her. She was allowed to place one of the colors anywhere on the paper. She was told (with the second color) that she could place the second color only in an empty space. She had to point to that empty space before putting the paint-laden brush there. While she was working I would say, "*Find* the empty space, *point* to the empty space, *paint in* the empty space. Your *eyes* are moving the brush." Anna began to separate her colors. She began to develop eye-hand coordination in a painless, non-threatened way. This did not happen overnight—it took a long time.

I found that Anna could not work with the Frostig program because not only did it require the use of a pencil or a crayon, but each diagram on every page posed too great a problem or threat to her. The drawings often look like those in a coloring book and are too tight and controlled to cope with. Anna's frustration grew whenever she was presented with this type of problem. Anna visibly began to impose her own self-controls when she was ready for them. And at that time we started behavior modification. When she needed to build her own controls, we gave her the painting exercises. Now when we put on music, Anna is more able to focus in on herself, create her own dance steps, and move her body rhythmically rather than erratically. She also builds with clay. She is beginning to form and to mold the clay in specific creations. What has happened is that this child—who at one time totally lacked eye-hand coordination—now can sit, look at the clay, and *make her hands work with her eyes* to successfully create forms that please her.

Theresa

Theresa spends most of her time with Mrs. S.'s class. Her behavior has improved in that she is able to control her acting-out behavior.

Early in the program Theresa had a score of 28 on the Peabody Picture Vocabulary Test. Her receptive language skills were greater than her expressive language. The last psychological work-up from her other school stated that she has "expressive aphasia." After spending much time with Theresa, I began to feel that there might also be a hearing problem. At my suggestion, she had a work-up done at a local hospital. The tests indicated partial deafness in one ear and almost complete deafness in the other ear. She is now wearing a hearing aid.

In the beginning, the group proved extremely beneficial for Theresa. By encouraging her to draw a good deal of the time, I allowed her to exhaust her theme of doctors, nurses and hospitals. Now she draws flowers and people—me, Mrs. S., and her friends in the class. Theresa is developing good peer relationships, her work is very high level, and she is happy. I feel good about what has happened to Theresa and I guess I find it hard to think of myself in a less important role for her now. It is difficult for me that she is beginning to relate to Mrs. S. more and more. Theresa no longer needs the dependency she had with me. I've tried to be very careful not to hold her back and I feel she has made a good transition. She is beautiful—she has grown—I think she is going to make it.

I asked Mrs. S. to write a short statement about Theresa. She writes: *Theresa has been participating in a structured, academically-oriented program, with a group of 10 youngsters, every morning for the last few months. She follows directions eagerly and well. She responds to praise as a flower to sunshine. She gets along very well with the youngsters in the group. She likes them and they are very fond of her. She recognizes capital letters and small letters of the alphabet. Her number concepts are fairly good—and she could use more work with the calendar. Theresa can and does function independently and imaginatively. She understands several directions without teacher supervision.*

Clara

Clara—sometimes I want to cradle you in my arms, sometimes I want to smack you. But most of the time you're sweet, lovable, and you make me think of myself. I see and feel your self-rejection and your wanting to hurt yourself. Your family makes unrealistic demands of you. They have expectations beyond your capabilities. They want

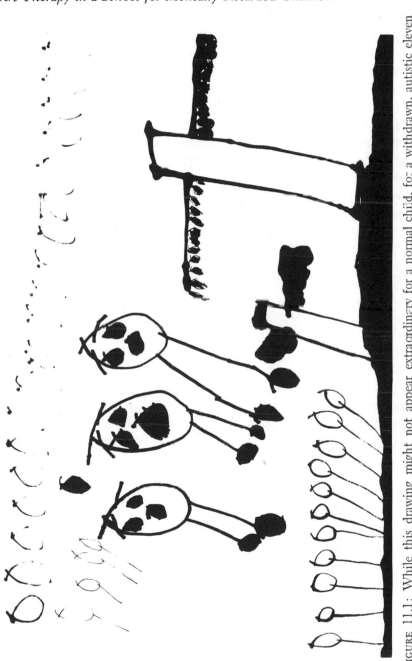
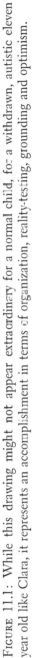

Figure 11.1: While this drawing might not appear extraordinary for a normal child, for a withdrawn, autistic eleven year old like Clara, it represents an accomplishment in terms of organization, reality-testing, grounding and optimism.

you to be a "normal" child. But I wonder, even if you were "normal," would you then be good enough for them? I don't think so. My family, too, was never satisfied with my achievements, nor did they recognize my abilities. And so, like you, Clara, I tended to remain infantile. When we went on the trip to the dental clinic and spent part of the time in the "apartment set-up," you went to the baby in the crib and held and fondled it. There was no destructive behavior. You treated the baby doll the way you want to be treated—with care and love and acceptance. It is so unfortunate that your family cannot see the sweetness and joy inside of you. You play and laugh, and it is so easy to see the goodness within you.

Clara's behavior has changed somewhat. Although she still may act on impulse, at least she has begun to feel a sense of herself (see Figure 11.1). To encourage this we've continually created situations that have emphasized her as a necessary and important part of our group. There are evidences of positive growth. Clara has experienced success in her work. She has been allowed and encouraged to express emotion; she is allowed to cry. When she does strike out uncontrollably I try to get her to verbalize what has happened. Just recently, I've tried to put more pressure on her in terms of her exerting greater controls over her impulsive behavior. She cries, but she also says, "I will try harder." So far she has. She lashed out at Anna one day. In a fit of frustration I hit her hand. I told her how upset I was with her for hitting Anna and with myself for hitting her. I said that maybe we can try to press our hands together when we feel like lashing out. Maybe we can tell each other what is bothering us.

Ellen

Ellen does not exhibit autistic, unresponsive behavior anymore. She does not do very much in the way of art work, but she will work with pegs, following a sequence of pattern. She has begun to lace. She can sort colors and shapes easily. She has recently begun to build with the large kindergarten blocks by herself. Ellen loves to brush her hair while admiring herself in the big mirror.

Her development to this point was very slow and much of her behavior was still infantile. She wanted everything done for her. As she became more and more responsive I began to place more and more pressure on her—one step at a time. She even pushed me away once—without withdrawing—and said, "No!" Her earlier one-word responses are now growing into short phrases and sometimes sentences. She usually does not verbalize much spontaneously. We keep taking slides of the girls and showing them. With Ellen's responsiveness to behavior modification, her vocabulary is slowly increasing. With the slides, she jumps up and points to what she recognizes.

Ellen had a cleft-palate operation at a very early age and this has caused speech problems for her. She seems to have poorly developed tongue and mouth muscles. She does not meet the requirements of the speech department in respect to the minimum Peabody score and they will not work with her. Since the speech department chooses not to be involved, we are giving her exercises to do. We tape a tissue on her nose and she has to blow it. She also blows bubbles through a bubble pipe. Ellen is putting forth a tremendous effort. She really wants to speak well, and she works hard at exercises and pronunciations.

Ellen dances with us now, although her movements are still somewhat stiff. She tries to bend her knees and swing her arms. She will move with me or my aide rather than push us away. The more Ellen relates to us and other people, the less frustrated she seems. She smiles and laughs frequently now.

Working with the Institution

Everything was going very smoothly until the administration decided to set up a new program in the senior department. They put together a group of five senior-age students who are severely retarded and who have been contained but not helped by the school for years. The administration finally decided that we were no longer to be simply babysitters for this group. And so a decision was made to use operant conditioning with them. The teacher's aide who had worked with me all those months was put in this new set-up. I was not told of this plan but found out about it on Friday when the move was to take place on the next Monday. I discussed the loss of my aide with my principal, who said he knew nothing about it. He had told the two assistant principals to place an aide in that group but did not know Helen (my aide) was going to be chosen. I complained about the continuing lack of professionalism—how no one gave me the courtesy of informing me of such a move or even consulting with me on it. Helen was upset and cried, and I was simply furious.

I won't go into the "politics" that have resulted in the replacement of Helen with Linda. Helen is an older woman who is physically large. She is a warm, smiling, loving, fondling mother figure. She was a good balance for me. All the children responded beautifully to her—especially Sharon. Helen was a very important figure for her. She would always comb Sharon's hair and put ribbons in it. She represented the large loving mother for all of us! My upset about this move was totally justified. Did they care about the relationship that was taking place between Helen, myself and the girls? I knew the girls would be able to adjust to the change eventually, but I worried most of all about Sharon. Helen was there when my strength ran out. When I worked through conflicts with Theresa and Clara, Helen was the warmth Sharon knew. She handled the class when a substitute was in. She loved the girls.

The new aide is a little younger than I am. For a while Linda found it very hard to work with me, and vice versa. She seemed to lack the spontaneity that Helen had. She could not get physically close to the girls for a long time. She had worked in structured classrooms where her job was spelled out for her. It was difficult for her when I would not give her a program to follow or a set of jobs to do. I would not establish a structure for her. For a while we were not happy working with each other. I resented her for taking Helen's place. She resented me for not giving her a structure to work within. I finally sat down with her one day and we talked out our feelings. From that time on, we both exerted greater effort towards making the situation work. I'm glad to say Linda's been working out beautifully. She has begun to understand the necessity of this type of program. She can now begin to see how it helps work through the changes that have taken place within the girls. She has good intuition. She, too, takes over when a substitute is in. She has been able to get physically close to the girls. For a long time the change was very hard for Sharon. She has now grown to like Linda and feel comfortable with her. But Linda cannot be that big, warm mother figure that Helen was any more than I can.

Linda and I have continued the shower program. We get undressed and get in there with the girls. They are learning how to wash their hair by themselves. The girls also go to a grooming class which is like a beauty parlor set-up. This is good, but I feel it is more important for them to learn to wash and brush their own hair.

Sharon

Sharon—my enigma. I feel like I want to love you; sometimes it's hard, sometimes it's easy. When I yell at you I hate myself for it, but you are my greatest source of frustration. One Friday morning during a language lesson, Sharon began talking to her fingers, rolling her eyes and breathing deeply. After watching this for a few minutes and feeling I could stand it no longer, I mirrored her. I imitated every movement she made. The more I imitated her, the more she continued the behavior. She was almost reaching a point of hysterical laughter, when I stopped mimicking her and took her over to "her" corner. Her corner is an area in the room next to the sink. It has a long mirror on the wall. I put a desk and chair in front of the mirror and a three-sided screen around the desk. Sharon talked to her fingers and went off into her fantasy world which is a secure non-threatening place. My reason for setting up the screen and desk is to give her an external sense of security. She needs to have a place where she can close herself off and be comfortable. This private place is where she was able to look at herself in the mirror and to relate to her own reflection. Then, as she began to talk to the reflection, she was able to *talk out* for the first time —rather than going completely inward. What she said sounded like a broken record or a tape that had not been edited. But that didn't matter. What mattered was that some of that stuff inside began to come out. Since then, she has gone to her corner frequently and just talks to herself in the mirror.

Recently I put Sharon on a behavior modification program to reinforce her verbalization. The behavior we worked on was to get her to say "Hello Ellis" after I said "Hello Sharon." As I said "Hello Sharon," I put my hand on her shoulder. As I had her repeat "Hello Ellis," I helped her move her hand to touch me. The reason for this was to begin to physically draw her away from herself and make appropriate physical contact with me. Most of the time now, she will say "Hello Ellis" after I say "Hello Sharon." She is slowly beginning to relate to some other people—Linda, Mrs. B., Mr. S. She may not always include the word "hello" but she will say their name rather than repeat what they say to her.

Last week Sharon had her period. She was cranky, crying, and not acting at all herself. She wore the same smelly, dirty clothes every day. Her body needed to be cleaned. Her mother does not seem to believe in taking a bath or shower during menstruation. I remember the horrendous menstrual pain I had when I was her age. I remember how difficult it was for me to accept menstruation as a natural function. Sharon is experiencing all of the internal changes and feelings of growing and she doesn't understand it.

Sharon is at a symbiotic level of relating. I remember lying down on the floor one afternoon as a result of complete exhaustion. My arms were out. Sharon crawled next to me, smiled, and placed her head under my arm. It felt as though an infant were crawling next to me and leaning on me for total support. Sharon had a traumatic experience related to her symbiotic needs while working with the puppets. The puppetry was started after someone in my supervision group suggested that I use this technique with Robin. I worked with Robin, Linda worked with Sharon and my Friday volunteer worked with the rest of the girls. I was unable to get any dialogue going with Robin. Linda worked with Sharon using the father and baby puppets. Sharon began playing with the baby puppet by herself. She didn't want to sit with Linda. She heard me with Robin and repeated some of what I was saying. A few minutes later Sharon ran from Linda. Linda tried to get her to sit but she wouldn't. Linda began a dialogue about the father and baby eating breakfast together. Sharon sat and listened. Then Linda showed the father hitting the baby puppet. Sharon screamed and ran away. She squeezed the baby puppet's face in. She took the puppet off and squished it in her hands. I went over to try and calm her. When I walked over to her she threw herself on the floor. Linda and the volunteer moved the girls to the other side of the room while Sharon threw her first full-fledged tantrum. She kicked me, cried, squirmed around. I didn't feel that she was just acting out. I was not going to mirror her now. She was experiencing physical changes that she could not understand. She reacted strongly to the puppets and the negative dialogue.

Sharon views me as a mother-figure and there I was with Robin—not with her—using mother and daughter puppets. When Linda tried to create a family situation, the shifting roles upset Sharon terribly. Sharon was not getting my attention. She saw me and heard the dialogue of a mother relating to a daughter. I noticed her watching me with a look of jealousy and contempt. I let her kick and scream. I spoke softly to her telling her it was all right. After a while she calmed down, held the baby puppet, and kissed it. We went over to the clay bin and we squeezed the clay in our fingers. The harder she squeezed it and the more she threw it, the bigger grew her smile. She wanted the puppets near her on the desk. She put the father, baby, and mother puppet right next to each other. She showed the father puppet kissing the baby puppet. Sharon's father is an old-fashioned, old-country Greek. He rejects her not only as a female, but as a female with a severe handicap. He has very little contact with her. After a while she put the puppets in their box and built with the clay.

During a conference with me, Sharon's mother said that her husband works hard and will not bother with the children and their school. She also says that when she took Sharon to a church in Greece years ago, she knew a miracle would eventually take place because the "sun shone on her as they walked up the steps." She believes that Sharon's handicap is a temporary "condition" and that someday Sharon will be able to marry and have children.

Today we washed and set Sharon's hair. We put lipstick and perfume on her. Today she is happy and says "Hello Ellis," "Hello Linda." Today she sits for twenty minutes with Ellen and both girls give appropriate verbal responses to the Peabody picture cards.

Looking Ahead

We have all experienced so much together this year. The girls have grown and so have I. Many of my old feelings still remain. I still have a sensitive overreaction when some of the other teachers with higher functioning students look at my group with disgust. We went on a trip to see *Sound of Music* with the entire elementary department. Many of the high-level academically-oriented students taught by "structured" teachers were yelling, jumping up and down, and behaving inappropriately. Miss Ellis' horribles sat, enjoyed the film, and behaved beautifully. I felt like Henry Higgins shepherding a flock of Eliza Doolittles to the ball. By George, they did it!

I worry about what will happen to them next year. I've written a proposal asking that I be allowed to run an art therapy program. I don't feel it is necessary to work with the same group all day long. I've asked for a set-up that would allow different children to come in at different times of the day and week. The proposal is still waiting to be discussed. I find it disturbing to consider the girls' future. There will be no problem finding an appropriate class placement for Theresa. I can think of one good placement for Clara, but that teacher has a full class. I have no other suggestions.

I can think of no other teacher, working with the age range of my girls, who would continue with them from the point where they are now. Teachers often stay with the same age-level children because of a certain degree of insecurity. I too am guilty of that. My girls have come from many of these teachers—I can't see them going back to them. I know it is up to the administration to find appropriate placements for students upon recommendations by the teacher, social worker, psychologist, and others. But when there isn't anyone appropriate—what happens? I would think that people would have to continually be trained to work with children who constantly pose new and different problems.

I am frustrated but it's not my problem alone to work out. I don't feel I should keep the girls because of a lack of appropriate placements. Whatever decisions are made will have to be done jointly. My girls exhibit behaviors that are different and therefore become a threat to some of the teaching staff. My own behavior for the last seven years has certainly not been one of a conformist. I've also been a threat to some of the people there.

I feel very positively (maybe foolishly) about the administration's acceptance of my proposal. I think the problems—the resentment and non-acceptance—will come from some of the staff. After all, isn't art therapy simply playing around? Those people who complain that my girls do nothing but play all day have been invited openly to see and discuss the program. No one has yet come!

Editor's note—After this report was written, Joan's proposal for setting up an art therapy program for "problem children" was accepted by the administration of the school in which she works. It is now in its second successful year.

COMMENTARY

The poetic rhythm of Joan's interaction is loud and clear: We hear the beat and song of her class throughout this report. Joan's approach illustrates the creative use of self in dealing with a complex and overwhelming group structure. Her responsiveness seems so free and unbounded that one wonders out loud. She must be spinning from all that is happening around her. But as one reads carefully, one finds that Joan's responsiveness and freedom are intermixed with a discipline that has come from a good deal of hard work and study. Indeed, far from being chaotic, the classroom atmosphere has a sense of purposefulness as Joan moves in and uses herself, attempting to relate uniquely to each child's maturational needs.

Art therapy in this particular context is not simply a matter of freeing a child's creative potential. There are sensory and perceptual needs that have long been neglected. Ego skills of these children are weak and shaky. Controls are needed with some; integration and reinforcement of adaptive patterns are needed for others.

All too often, behavior modification techniques are utilized in classroom situations in a dehumanized and sterile manner. In this particular instance, this is very far from the case. Thus, each child not only internalizes a more functional and adaptive pattern through reinforcement, but also takes in a rich and loving model that will build the self with care rather than with rigidity and sterility.

At the other end of the continuum, we see Joan utilizing sensory-awareness techniques. She plays, feels, and touches with each child so that there can be a greater awareness of one's body-self. Again this approach is integrated within a framework that is neither rigid nor chaotic. Joan is concerned with creativity development and the expansion of self. In order to accomplish these goals, she must respond to a number of maturational deficiencies that are so clearly in evidence. She holds and mirrors; she reacts and receives; she allows herself to be close and yet makes a distance. In a word, she is the mother lioness setting the basis for a strong ego so that the self can be free. But this mother lion does not confine herself to the den. She attempts to relate to the community, the school institution, and, where possible, the family. This is art therapy in its true humanistic tradition.

12. Art Therapy as an Experience with a Schizophrenic Child

Susan Mann

INTRODUCTION

I am imagining myself as the Jeremy that Susan describes. I feel very small, even one-dimensional. I cannot separate me from the room I am in. . . . I am bombarded by colors, sounds, scents; afraid of being gobbled up by everything around; obsessed with whooshing myself away to see what remains. People are no different from toilets and floor waxers—they move suddenly and powerfully: They consume me in a whirling rush.

Susan and the art work seem to offer just the amount of contact he can take without vanishing. He uses both to control his environment, to select his input, to create, manipulate, destroy, and recreate, rather than having it all done to him. Though at first she senses that he needs her entirely to perform these feats, Susan also remains distant—or more precisely, she remains parallel to him at this point. She accepts being an appendage, an unobtrusive presence, another machine—not an overwhelming one, for once, but smooth-running, quiet, no sudden starts, no breakdowns, just working at the touch of Jeremy's hand.

As Jeremy merges and emerges, Susan stays parallel and constant. Her presence seems to remind him that he is still there. She seems to sense that this child would be devastated by overprotective arms reaching out, smothering, making him disappear into darkness. Jeremy can begin to notice Susan because she does not overwhelm him—she's manageable, she speaks softly when everything else roars. She is steady, does not allow him to lose himself, subtly begins to bargain for new steps: I'll do this . . . now you do that . . . you *can* do that. . . . Watch how we make this little machine . . . now watch how you place the switch . . . no electric shocks, no fireworks; you and I are still here.

Jeremy responds and emerges through art, I think, because it is a

144

safe opportunity to relate to his non-human environment—first passively, then more actively. Next, it seems to become a transitional object—I guess Susan could then be called the transitional subject—which allows tentative expression of needs and fears. Finally, the art work helps develop safe familiar patterns which gradually change and challenge through Susan's careful monitoring.

THE CASE—JEREMY

Two days a week I work in a therapeutic nursery classroom. The classroom is a therapeutic setting for four severely disturbed preschool
children, all males, most of whom may be described as exhibiting
various forms of early childhood psychosis. The children attend the
nursery five days a week for about five hours each day. Their activities
are supervised by two teacher-therapists who attempt to create with
the children a stimulating and nurturing environment where they will
have the opportunity to learn to interact with their teacher-therapists
and each other in a meaningful way. It is hoped that, in this environment, the children will be helped to acquire basic skills that will enable them to function more effectively and independently and perhaps
even be able to enter a more normal setting after their nursery experience. The environment is a very supportive one where the children
are frequently rewarded for acceptable behavior with praise and acceptance and reprimanded with clear and direct statements indicating
why the behavior is inappropriate.

For the past three months I have been spending at least a portion of
my days at the nursery with Jeremy, a four-year-old schizophrenic
child. I do not have a great deal of information about Jeremy's background. I do know that his parents are divorced and that he lives with
his mother and grandmother. As the parents were separated before
Jeremy's birth, he has never really known a male figure in the household. Jeremy is a very beautiful child, small and delicate in appearance,
and, although his motor coordination is below normal, he gives the
feeling of being quite graceful. He exhibits many of the characteristics
common to early childhood schizophrenia: an insensitivity to pain,
failure to have developed adequate speech, paying more attention to
objects than to people, a difficulty in playing with other children, a
hypersensitivity to loud sounds, abnormal fears and also a lack of an
appropriate sense of fear, and, in most areas, a short attention span.
Also, he has a tendency to withdraw into himself, especially when demands are placed on him—it is often difficult to elicit his cooperation
in fulfilling such demands as sitting at the table long enough to finish
his lunch.

Although Jeremy's attention span is usually very limited, he is incredibly responsive to art activities and often is content to paint or
play with clay for anywhere from 15 to 30 minutes, becoming quite

agitated if we have to end the session before he is ready. Also, the things that we create in these art sessions are very important to him, and he likes to keep his paintings or clay objects with him for the rest of the day. If that is not possible, then he at least likes to know exactly where they are and will check them out at various times during the day.

When I first met Jeremy he was quite obsessed with the idea of floor-waxers and would indiscriminately approach just about any adult entering the classroom with a plea to draw him a floor-waxer. I used this obsession as a launching point for our art sessions. It was arranged that I would work with Jeremy in a corner of the classroom which was physically set off from the rest of the room by a high cupboard and so afforded a certain amount of privacy from the other activities going on in the room. We began with my painting crude representations of floor-waxers for Jeremy with his guiding me by resting his hand on mine. He was already painting by himself in regular group painting sessions done earlier in the day before I arrived, but he seemed to be very fearful of trying to execute anything as highly-charged as a floor-waxer by himself. He would become so excited that he was virtually unable to manipulate the paintbrush in any controlled way. Also, he seemed to be very afraid of getting his hands dirtied by the paint. It should be mentioned that Jeremy's previous paintings did not appear to be in any way representational so that part of this excitement and confusion could be attributed to the fact that I was encouraging him for the first time to represent an emotion through a drawing. This can be highly-charged even for a normal child.

As Jeremy and I drew the floor-waxers, usually a multitude of them on any one piece of paper, I would attempt to explore his feelings with him by discussing what we were doing. Our discussions, however, were rather limited.

JEREMY: Draw a blue floor-waxer.
SUSAN: Susan will draw a blue floor-waxer. Jeremy can help Susan draw a blue floor-waxer.
JEREMY: Draw a red floor-waxer. Amazing!
SUSAN: Susan and Jeremy will draw a red floor-waxer. A floor-waxer is a machine. It is a machine used to clean floors.
JEREMY: Draw a blue floor-waxer. Make a switch! Make a switch!
SUSAN: Jeremy can make a switch. Here, Jeremy make a switch.

And so we would explore various aspects of a floor-waxer—that it is a machine, that it makes a loud noise, etc. I felt that it was important that Jeremy make his own switches so that, in addition to its being a way for him to participate more actively in the drawings, he could hopefully feel that he had control over the machines by having control over drawing the switches that turn them on and off. Gradually, during these sessions, Jeremy began to lean the full weight of his body on mine—he still continues to do so even now. This was the first way he allowed me to have physical contact with him.

During this time I was also experimenting with cut-outs of floor-waxers and vacuum-cleaners from colored-paper in order to encourage Jeremy to develop some independent play. This was fairly successful in that he would spend quite a bit of time moving them about in the air and on the floor. This particular play was usually done during nap-time—a period of time after lunch when we all attempt to relax.

About the same time we began to explore floor-waxers, Jeremy also began to behave compulsively towards the toilet. He would run into the bathroom very excitedly exclaiming he wanted to "make a sissy" and would frantically begin to flush the toilet. In the middle of this flushing, when you were able to get his pants down, he would attempt to urinate. He did this so often during the day that he seldom had much to urinate, but when he was finished he would stick his arms into the toilet-bowl and somehow again begin to flush. I feel that this toilet behavior closely parallels his obsession with floor-waxers. The actual act of pulling down Jeremy's pants gives him the opportunity to check out that his penis is there and intact. The toilet, when it is flushed, makes a loud noise and literally consumes the urine that came from Jeremy's penis. To Jeremy it must seem that this powerful noisy toilet might also eat up his penis or perhaps even Jeremy himself. This fear of being consumed also seems apparent in Jeremy's obsession with floor-waxers. A floor-waxer is also a loud machine which resembles the shape of a large penis—even down to having two brushes at the bottom as the testicles. All of the drawings made for Jeremy of floor-waxers looked just like crude representations of a penis and testicles, no matter how much we attempted to make them look more like actual floor-waxers. Jeremy's penis is surely no match for such a large machine-penis so that Jeremy could very likely fear that he would be destroyed by this large noisy machine. Jeremy at least can have some control over all of these machines by making sure they all have switches so that he can be assured of being able to turn them off. In fact, switches in general seem to generate a lot of fear in Jeremy. He becomes very fearful, for instance, when lights are switched off or on unexpectedly.

Jeremy's interest in cut-outs of floor-waxers prompted me to introduce clay to his play. At first he was very afraid of the clay as it probably too closely resembled feces. Also, as with the paint at first, he did not like having the clay dirty his hands. I brought in a clay floor-waxer which I had made at home. I explained that this was a *clay* floor-waxer. The waxer broke and, to Jeremy's surprise, we were able to fix it by mending the break with soft clay. After this we proceeded to make a few more waxers out of soft clay. Seeing the object already made from clay, then seeing how it could be made again from soft clay worked well as a nice transition. Jeremy learned that he could participate in making the floor-waxers with me when he stepped on one of the newly-made waxers and was able to bend the handle back into place by himself. Eventually, although I would actually make the parts of the waxer—a disk for the bottom and a shaft for the top— Jeremy would help me by pressing the two parts together. As with the paintings, it was Jeremy's job to include the switches. This he did by sticking one or many pieces of pipe cleaner or paper clips into the clay.

My long-range goals began to formulate about this time in Jeremy's play and seem to have remained pretty much the same. My objective became to work with Jeremy so that he could use both the paint and the clay without physically relying on me to construct or draw for him and so he would be able to recreate his experiences through art so that we could then discuss them. This does not mean that Jeremy should be able to paint or construct with any particular artistic skill— just that he be able to create something by himself.

The transition from my painting for Jeremy to his painting for himself came about the same day that another important development occurred. We had been to the gymnasium earlier in the day and Jeremy had been quite frightened by a large square piece of wood hanging by hinges from the wall. Another child had been banging this piece of wood against the wall and this made quite a loud and reverberating noise. Also, the same child had spent some time playing with a light-switch which controlled the red exit light over the door. Later, when we became involved in our art session, which this day involved painting, Jeremy asked me to draw him a gym. This was the first time that he had ever asked me to draw anything except floor-waxers and the occasional vacuum-cleaner. He then asked me to draw a big square

piece of wood which I did, and then I repeated drawing the squares as
Jeremy repeated the request until we had drawn four or five pieces of
wood. He then requested that I draw a red light. I replied that Jeremy
could draw the red light by himself which he did. We talked for some
time about Jeremy's frightening experiences in the gym and finally the
discussion reverted once again to the subject of floor-waxers. I encouraged Jeremy to draw the waxers by himself and for the first time he did
so without my assistance. So, for the first time, not only did he draw
by himself but he also brought into the art session a new experience—
one that had troubled him that very same day.

Jeremy continued drawing floor-waxers by himself for many weeks
and also continued to make many clay floor-waxers with my assistance.
He did not, however, bring any other new experiences into the sessions for some time. Finally it was decided that we should try to
encourage him not to draw or construct only floor-waxers. The transition occurred quite naturally in our sessions. By this time Jeremy was
requesting daily that we work in clay, and it was with clay that we
developed a pattern that we are still using now. The pattern involves
his requesting that I make him something—he is still afraid to actually
manipulate the clay himself—and then he plays with these things
while we talk about them. At first it was necessary to ignore most of
his requests for floor-waxers and explain to him that I wanted him to
make something else. I tried making egg beaters, birthday cakes, anything that related to his experiences during the day. Finally, Jeremy
seemed to get the idea and requested that we make a toilet. We
experimented with pieces of pipe cleaner and paper clips coming out
of a hole in the bottom of the toilet. He started also to experiment
with making his own machines which consist of free-form pieces of
clay into which he sticks paper clips, pipe-cleaners—anything that is
within reach that will fulfill his requirements for that particular machine. These free-form objects are just as real—if not more real—to
him than the objects that I make for him.

Jeremy's requests to date have expanded from frantic demands for
floor-waxers to more calm requests for other inanimate objects within
his experience. I have come now to include another goal in my hopes
for Jeremy—that is for him to include living things in his art experiences. I feel that he has been most responsive to art therapy, in part
because he is already such a willing subject when it comes to doing
anything involving art. The art sessions, however, provided me with a
much better understanding of Jeremy's progression which can be seen

so clearly through the development of his paintings and clay forms. For instance, now that Jeremy seems to have almost lost interest in drawing or making floor-waxers, he has also almost stopped compulsive behavior over the toilet. His expanded interest in drawing new experiences seems to parallel an expanded awareness of his environment which includes more intelligible speech, a greater awareness of the presence of his peers, and many other more subtle things. Jeremy is, of course, getting a great deal of support from many sources, but I believe that art has played a significant role in his development and will continue to do so.

COMMENTARY

Susan tentatively enters into Jeremy's world and makes contact through the vehicle of the "floor-waxer." She is careful not to overwhelm him and slowly allows his need for physical contact to manifest itself. Slowly, Jeremy senses that he will not be swallowed up by the therapist and lets his full weight lean on Susan. Thus, the initial foundation of building an ego is made. Without deep body contact, the very raw material of repairing or building an identity cannot proceed.

Observing both participants, one is impressed by the heavy concentration of ego-building skills that characterizes this relationship. Through the "switch," Susan encourages Jeremy to get some feeling of control. He can turn it on and off, control the noise and movement, and move backwards and forward. The ego skills of motility, integration, and initiative are all positively reinforced.

The use of cut-outs helps to extend his world. They are transitions from his original home-base—close enough for security, yet pointing outward rather than inward.

Susan broadens the ego's ability for mastery. Clay replicas of the waxer are made and repaired—a symbolic rebirth and regeneration of the self. Maybe life is not so full of danger and annihilation after all. Broken "things" can be repaired—so can trust. Of note is that the very foundations of creative expression are given some definition through creation and recreation of the clay floor-waxer.

The description of Jeremy's use of art therapy, as in his handling his fear of the large square piece of wood and the noises associated with it, illustrates some very basic principles of symbolic expression. Vague uncanny fears are objectified, concretized, and talked about. These are all steps for Jeremy in gaining some self-mastery.

Susan gives an extremely fine illustration of the functions of art therapy with schizophrenic children. Far from being concerned with the release of fantasy material, her preoccupation is one of building an ego with the help of art materials. At least two factors involved in creative expression must constantly be evaluated. Some children, as in the case of Jeremy, need to develop integrative skills to be able to communicate what is inside of them. Other patients may need a breakdown of inhibiting or restricting defenses in order to let the raw power of their fantasy emerge in a creative statement about themselves. The

art therapist must be a specialist not only in understanding unconscious processes, but also in perceiving the intricacies of ego organization. Jeremy will need much help in this area. He must master such
skills as motor-coordination, motility, judgment, reality testing, ob-
jectification in order to really make use of himself. Reinforcement
techniques are used by this therapist without the aura of a scientific
methodology. Art therapy is presented by Susan in a most dynamic
and sophisticated fashion. She is literally helping to build an identity
through art.

13. The Use of Film, Photography and Art with Ghetto Adolescents

Barbara Maciag

INTRODUCTION

Barbara has given us a veritable primer in working with ghetto children, adolescents, and street gang members. Many students have worked in this rather infamous area or one like it—but few have gotten as deeply into the inner workings of the people there or have been able to express so clearly what they have found.

Barbara's presence is important to understand. I once saw her dressed as Little Orphan Annie, and the comparison is not far off: She is as seemingly innocent and tiny of voice and body, as capable of taking care of herself, and as ageless. What often seems to be naïveté in her dealings is actually an incredible wealth of experience turned into practical understanding of what she, in fact, can handle. You could swear she's got a Daddy Warbucks somewhere for the way she walks into apparently difficult situations and turns them into simple, easily-handled experiences through common sense and mature straight-forwardness.

Barbara herself points out that her success with these street-gang adolescents is due to her gentleness and her lack of any need to compete with them or of any unreasonable fear. Her knowledge and love of her media—film, photography, art—and her quickly absorbed understanding of the reality of her people cannot be overlooked as additional contributing factors.

It would be impossible to highlight all the issues in her multi-dimensional report so I will remain with a few which were most meaningful to me. First, there was Barbara's perception of herself as being treated like a camera with her film group—and her discovery of their genuine acceptance of her when the camera broke. The feeling of hiding behind art techniques or of being treated as "just an art teacher" is quite common among fieldwork experiences. In my work with a disturbed man, I remember becoming more or less involved in intricate art work as our reflected anxieties increased or diminished. Sometimes this is a response to a client's feelings; sometimes it seems to be a necessary beginning or respite for both.

Barbara's clear distinction of when racial differences become a therapeutic issue and when they do not indicates a genuine acceptance of herself and her group members as individuals rather than as stereotypes. Her sophisticated understanding of drug abuse provides the foundation for a realistic approach which is geared appropriately to the setting.

Barbara also touches some tender inner issues. Her helplessness in dealing with a girl in her art group and the girl's psychotic mother is particularly poignant. Her ability to let-be and to allow her men to unfold through media they enjoy together is remarkable. The image which most touched me was that of her separation from a strong beautiful son in whose development she had participated. This shows Barbara's willingness to accept what she has meant to these people. Most of us find it much easier to accept what our clients have meant to us.

Finally, I would like to apply an issue which Dr. Robbins has mentioned—that some ghetto people are suspicious of therapists who have "made it" in this society. Barbara seems to represent the best of both worlds: She sacrifices neither the objective viewpoint and knowledge which come from good training nor the integrity and individual creativity in being an authentic individual.

THE CASE

History

I denote my three art therapy groups according to the media they preferred to use: film, art and photography. Below is additional information to help further differentiation.

Photography

This was my first art therapy group. We met for eight months at a community mental health center. Members built a darkroom to utilize the enlarger donated by a staff member, the center reimbursed me for supplies, and I lent my Canon FTb 35mm camera for the group's use. Members were most involved with photographing each other during our sessions, and occasionally their families, girlfriends, and girls passing on the streets. All members did their own developing and printing in our darkroom at the center. This group consisted of 12 Hispanic men, ages ranging between 13 and 23 years, some of whom belonged to various street gangs.

Art

We met for nine months at a public junior high school. Members used their sketchbooks as creative diaries to draw their fantasies, adventures, Winnicott "squiggles" and "Masterpieces" (graffetti names such as *Love Factory 186*, done in multicolor, or simply *Slick*) (see Figure 13.1). We were given our own room at the school on the walls of which the group painted murals as an artistic statement of themselves. There were two Hispanic and four Black non- or ex-gang members, including one female.

Film

This group consisted of an entire division of a large local street gang. We met for three months in their clubhouse to make a film of

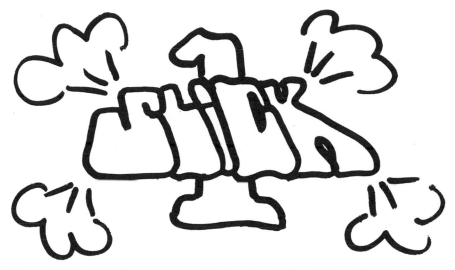

FIGURE 13.1: Graffiti names were developed and discarded rapidly in a phase-appropriate search for identity. SLICK 1's lettering resembles the slicks or tires of hotrods, a common phallic symbol for this adolescent group.

what it is to be a street gang member. I supplied the camera, they supplied the projector and screen, and the center reimbursed me for the film. This division consisted of approximately 15 Hispanic men in adolescence through the twenties.

Introduction

The purpose of this paper is to discern and investigate the singularities and similarities of the three groups described above. A pause to look back and sort out information and experiences can facilitate insight into old problems and more creative solutions to new ones. To look back is also a natural part of the mourning I am experiencing for my groups following termination. I feel as a mother would in the final separation from a son, not a baby but a strong and beautiful young man whose growth has been a profound experience to watch and sometimes to participate in. I feel enthusiastic at the prospect of developing my thoughts on these three groups into some kind of frame for future reference. I also feel reluctant to begin because it's kind of a eulogy and a very final thing.

Defenses and Countertransferences

Apart from a group, one's defenses loosen and permit insights to which one was impervious while actively perticipating in that group. An example involves Miguel from my photography group whom I related to primarily in terms of his extrapunitive behavior. At one point Miguel brusquely gave me an embroidered rose patch for my pants and later a leather necklace he made. On both occasions, my reaction was, "How sweet of Miguel, my monster, to do this for me," and then to take his gifts home proudly and hang them up on my bulletin board. It did not occur to me until six months later that these were sensual objects which Miguel had probably visualized my utilizing and not hanging up on my bulletin board. I used to be a great blocker when it came to sex. I am now much more relaxed in dealing with sexual material—and feel it is important for sexually repressed and confused young men to experience a calm response to their sexuality.

The individual from whom I learned the most, because he made me learn the most about myself, was Ramon (Photography). I didn't realize how much alike we were until I had begun my own therapy and, in groping for a way to get something into focus, repeatedly heard myself saying, "Well, it's like what happened with Ramon when. . . ."

I myself began to experience Ramon's fear of closeness—of having experienced defensive isolation for so long and now having to decide to open up to the possibility of yet another hurt for the chance to experience love—which, coupled with self-disclosure, might even lead to self-love.

After missing a session, Ramon showed up and remarked in a surly way that I "should feel lucky that he was there." I instinctively replied, "And you should feel lucky that I'm here." Ramon summed up with, "Well, that's what I'm saying—you're lucky that I'm here and I'm lucky that you're here," denying the emotional commitment in our relationship of five months and making it a favor-being-given thing. When asked if I had fears of becoming dependent on her, I replied to my therapist, "Why, I hadn't even considered it. My attitude is that we're both just coming here with a job to do," fiendishly denying the warm attachment I felt towards her. I am reminded of the sign Ramon made and hung on the door to our workroom, "*Danger Watch Out*" in big warning letters. And I now realize just what that sign meant to him, although I couldn't express it then.

In addition to my continued therapy, Bruno Bettelheim's book, *Truants From Life* (1)—in particular the case study of Paul—was very helpful in understanding the dynamics of the relationship between Ramon and me. Some of the trials Paul felt obliged to put his therapist through before their relationship could flourish made Ramon look like a lamb. Anything of Bettelheim's that I've read, especially *Symbolic Wounds* (2), *Puberty Rites and the Envious Male* (3) and even his articles in the *Ladies Home Journal,* has given me a more profound understanding of the young people I work with.

The Day the Camera Broke and I Found Out I Was a Person

When I first began working with the street gang, I know I defensively related to them as an extension of the camera. I felt it was an ideal situation to meet in their clubhouse, but I also felt overwhelmed by the quantity of new stimuli and I figured I'd peek out at it from behind the one thing that was familiar to me. Hector, who instigated my being there, insured that my presence would be acceptable to the group. I liked them and enjoyed being there, but had only paranoid speculations as to how they felt about me. Every session, as soon as the filming was completed, I'd leave. Then one grim day we projected a new roll of film which should have been a masterpiece, and it came out disappointingly dark. Next we created a perfect lighting set-up, only to find that a gear had worn through in the camera. I had nothing to hide behind and had been at that session too short a time to feel good about leaving. By staying a while, I was able to realize it was only my fantasy that I was hidden behind a camera. The gang had been relating to me as a person all along—a person of whom they were quite fond, incidently—and their tolerance for disappointment and anxiety was greater than mine. This they helped me to cope with in their therapeutic manner—offering me a cigarette (they smoke, I don't, but made an exception this time) and engaging me in a friendly conversation that made me feel very much with them. We've since had a mutually satisfying relationship, and I felt really relieved at discovering that I had been a person to them all along.

I utilized a similar defense with my photography group. When told what my fieldwork assignment was—an experience which included working in a darkroom with adolescent men—many a listener's communication, verbal or otherwise, would be, "Boy, are you gonna get it now." When I didn't "get it" or even feel threatened, but instead happy and comfortable, I incredibly associated this with the fact that I wore blue jeans. Only girls who wear dresses must "get it."

After a few months Ramon, who had an unconscious genius for uncovering my every defense, commented, "Some people think that girls who never wear dresses are dykes. . . ." I assumed he was referring to me, worried that I was providing a negative female model, braced myself and wore a dress (after discreetly waiting a few sessions). Of course no one related to me any differently because I had been a female to them all along—wearing a dress hardly changed that and only one person even said, "Barbara, you have a dress on today."

Reality testing can be such a chore. But I also feel that my defensive behavior in these situations was prompted by a defensive need in the people I was relating to, and that when I was motivated to change it was because of a mutual growth in our relationship.

Of course I was a person to the street gang, but they probably found it hard to believe that I was interested in them other than filmically. Their transference made me feel like a camera with them until that line of communication temporarily broke down and we found the relationship could continue without a camera.

My photography group, Ramon in particular, had many conflicts about their sexuality and about relating successfully to the opposite sex. Their anxiety about self-control with women had me feeling that to be a neuter was the only way we could be comfortable together. Ramon's challenge to me to wear a dress was a symbolic test of our relationship to withstand our assorted rape fantasies should he relate to me as a woman.

Dr. Searles' book, *The Nonhuman Environment* (4), helped me to be aware of how a patient's transference can team up with a therapist's anxieties to create such defensive behavior in the therapist.

Females in El Barrio

You may wonder, as I did, why I have worked with approximately 40 men and one female. As much as it is considered a macho thing for many of the young men I've worked with to hang loose and act out, many of the "nice" females are thoroughly repressed, being let out of the house only for school and occasional grocery shopping until they are engaged. When I try to discuss the unfairness of this with the men they reply, "I wouldn't want my sister to be out on these streets." But even were they to be given a choice, many girls seem only to see their future security in the self-perpetuating cycle of ghetto poverty and defeatism—persuading a guy to drop out of school with her and marry to escape a smothering and unfulfilling home life, having a baby immediately to keep her company while her trapped young man takes to the streets, then lots of babies to smother-love in place of her errant husband (scc Figure 13.2).

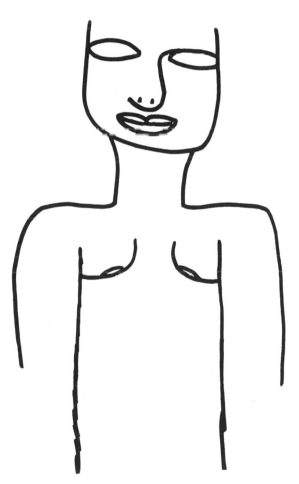

FIGURE 13.2: Although capable of more sophisticated images, some female adolescents produced figures of ambiguous gender. Perhaps the drawing reflects the phase-specific task of coming to terms with bisexuality and an acceptance of the passive, receptive female attitude.

Unless he has some group, such as a street gang or social club, in which it is possible to develop one's self-esteem, the ghetto man is generally made to feel helpless and hopeless by his environment. Acquiring a woman becomes important to his self-image, as offspring become living proof of his masculinity. But ghettos do not provide jobs, so a man's feelings of impotence and inadequacy are reinforced when he cannot support his family and is driven to less socially oriented behavior to survive. Overcrowded schools and centers attend to the troublesome act-outer—males almost by definition—and leave the withdrawers be, which is another reason why the groups I worked with are predominantly male. If a female does act out, it is usually sexually, and this seems to merit ostracization, not therapy, in the community.

So I work with what I have—being something of a novelty, unmarried at 23 years of age—"no, nothing's wrong, I just do not want to get tied down caring for a baby right now . . ." I can at least present another alternative that may not have been considered because of the overwhelming pressure in one direction. Channel 13's *Realidades* did a program on Puerto Rican men going in the armed forces at the time of the Vietnamese conflict.

> INTERVIEWER: Are you going in?
> PUERTO RICAN MAN: Yeah, there's nothing for me on these streets . . . same hanging out, hustling. In the army they told me I could sign up to be a medic, then when I get out I could get a job as a nurse, work in a hospital.
> INTERVIEWER: What about dropping bombs on people, is that going to bother you at all? Or getting hit yourself?
> PUERTO RICAN MAN: I hadn't thought about that at all. I think I've made the right decision for myself.

Race

After I made my presentation for Dr. Robbins' Advanced Seminar in Art Therapy, someone commented on the fact that I am White, working exclusively with Non-whites (sic) and how did I deal with that?—and that they would have said right at the beginning, "Look, I know that I'm White and you're not but I think it's a lousy system too, etc . . ."

I know that I'm not a very verbally aggressive person, but this approach instinctively turned me off. First, why should anyone believe you? Second, I don't feel as though I have to apologize for being White. I am what I am. People's eyes communicate more profoundly than the color of their skin.

As Lorraine Hansberry made clear to us in *To Be Young, Gifted and Black* (5), it isn't a matter of race at all—race is just the current manifestation of the much broader issue of how man has always persecuted his fellow man. Other centuries and cultures had different manifestations of the same condition. But this does not mean that because we know that it is not really a matter of race, that we can afford not to deal with race. As long as people are being persecuted or feel persecuted because of race, it must be a matter of concern to any therapist. When Frankie (Art) looks in the mirror when he's on LSD and sees himself with a paleface, then race becomes an important element in our therapy—not when he walks in the room and sees a White art therapist. I do feel that it is important for people to have a choice—that a Black therapist should be had if that's what's important. But I feel that it is equally vital for an individual to know that he can have a meaningful and therapeutic relationship with another human being, no matter what his race.

When I first worked with people who still feel close to their Puerto Rican homeland, I was very aware of entering a different culture. I found this challenging, fascinating, and exciting, and have sought to gain insight into the Puerto Rican-American perspective. I feel one can go only so far unless one has a grasp of the cultural orientation of the person one is working with. Literature on the contemporary Puerto Rican-American is, to my knowledge, rather sparse. My most accurate and immediate source is the people themselves, their homes, streets, botanicas, music and bodegas. For a broader perspective, I recommend Channel 13's *Realidades*. I have found that program to be consistent with my experience. I have found the treatment of street gangs by most of the mass media to be smacking of sensationalism and titillation with a careless misunderstanding or lack of insight into the Puerto Rican culture.

My young group members' fantasies of me do not seem to contain race and culture as critical elements. I am reminded of the time Miguel came to visit after having left the group for a month and began speaking to me in Spanish. I stared at him with a blank look until he said, "Barbara, that's right, you don't speak Spanish, do you?"

Milagros (Art) is working on a way for me to roll up my hair so I can have a six-foot Afro. These groups seem more concerned with establishing how alike we are, and even in the two examples I've given defining our differences, it is done mistakenly or in play. I feel this is more because of an understanding on this level than repression. I have dealt intensively with race in the course of my employment as a graphic designer for a Black community college. I have found that when people mature within a segregated group, they are more likely to attribute bizarre qualities to members of the out group, for various reasons, as described by Allport in *The Nature of Prejudice* (6).

Parents

Each group seems to have its own way of relating to parents. My "artists" are generally eager to have me come to their homes and meet their families. They still seem to take their identity from the family and to feel secure about my seeing them in family interactions, no matter how pathological they might be. Frankie first motivated me to include parents in my experience of an individual by bringing his mother to one of our first sessions. This experience was so pleasurable and interesting, I decided to meet other parents when a group member presented me with an opportunity to do so.

Milagros' mother (a psychotic junkie, I found out the hard way) prompted me to make a home-visit by drawing in Milagros' therapy sketchbook a series of shockingly hellish pencil sketches which Milagros told me were family crests. Milagros had been exhibiting increased psychotic symptoms and my "class" was the only one she was attending, otherwise wandering the halls of the school the rest of the week and telling her teachers she was with me. Her harried guidance counselor saw the solution as forbidding Milagros to continue with me, feeling this would get her to attend her classes. Milagros and I, in our divergent ways, were very upset by this decision, and I requested family therapy for Milagros with an empathic psychiatric social worker from the center with which I am affiliated. As usual, everything got bogged down in red tape—the Child Welfare Board wouldn't become involved because the last time a worker went there ten months ago, he got mugged in their building. Milagros' mother's welfare status gets threatened because of child neglect and a general freakout occurs.

Angela, Milagros' mother, is so well-read and intelligent that—were she ever able to get herself together—I am confident she would prove comparable to William Burroughs, who clearly established in his brilliant and bitter *Naked Lunch* (7) that not just dopes are on dope. What to do? Back off from the red-tape route which, at best for Angela, will probably result in further bitterness, isolation and fantasy or incarceration in a psychiatric ward of a charming local hospital? Just what real therapeutic help is available to someone in this ghetto who hasn't got MONEY and who is too in despair, too intelligent or too proud to assert herself at the few inadequate facilities available?

I do not feel comfortable in the Messiah role Milagros and Angela indicate they would like to see me in. Yet I have no confidence in the institutions and agencies accessible to these people. The places I would recommend are absurdly expensive with the average stay a lengthy one. Otherwise I usually have more confidence in an individual's capacity for self-healing with therapeutic help from a friend. So do I give time I don't have to give to talk and draw with Milagros and Angela because they have chosen me and I responded to a point?

I visit homes particularly with this group because they are the youngest and least likely to work through problems independently. For example, it is the (untherapeutic, I feel) policy of their school to transfer pupils to a local reform school for a couple of months when they exhibit behavior the school feels it cannot deal with—most notably the young men's hitting or "feeling up" female students. Coincidentally, students are given no sex education. I don't enjoy feeling cut off from a group member and do not want him to feel abandoned by the group. My art group is especially self-disclosing and it seems too precious an experience to be arbitrarily interrupted. Since I work with the "troublemakers," my group would be in quite a state of flux if we didn't develop a way of coping with this situation. At my request, both schools have agreed to let the students return for our art therapy sessions. That the students make the trek back confirms my position on this matter. When a transfer occurs, I visit at home to tell the family what a valuable group member their young man is because, more often than not, he is also the family scapegoat and his transfer serves to reinforce this role. Seeing the family interactions of my group member and the manner in which family members relate to me is always of value to further my understanding of the individual, as well as hopefully enhancing his position in the family.

On the other hand, my photography men, who were older, rarely mentioned their home lives. They seemed to want to break away and make a separate identity for themselves, but the lack of jobs in El Barrio hardly made this feasible. They utilized isolation and fantasy as defenses against their disturbing home environments and were involved with presenting themselves to me almost as self-made myths. I felt it would be too penetrating to enter their real worlds until our relationship became more balanced with reality. As long as they were into it, I felt it to be just as valid for me to hear what they would like to be as to know what they really were.

With my film group I have two families per person to relate to—their immediate family and the extended family of the street gang. I feel most everyone belongs to the club because of the inability of his immediate family to satisfy his basic emotional needs. This occurs in all the groups I work with, but the club provides a viable alternative to its members. The basement apartment clubhouse is received in exchange for maintenance of the above building. It is always a comfortable refuge—when there is no place else to go—with a dark, womb-like interior with mystical day-glo paintings gleaming under a black light. There are well-defined rules, procedures, and attitudes (similar in scope, but not content, to a religious order such as the Black Muslims) consistently enforced by the most creative father-figures of the ghetto—the clique presidents.

With one exception, I've experienced the five presidents I have known as intelligent, skillful, kind, charismatic leaders who are like resident therapists without vacation. The members demand more attention from them than one would from a father, and I often wondered just what was in it for the leaders—not much except the enormous responsibility and love I had anticipated and confirmed talking to Shep, an ex-president of the total membership of all this street gangs divisions.

I met Shep when I went to visit Milo, Shep's brother-in-law. Although I was accompanied by two young men, I had difficulty deciding whether or not to proceed when we turned onto Milo's block—the filth and decay were menacing, like a war-zone waiting for more bombs to be dropped, even in Milo's building. But as soon as one entered their apartment, it was a different world—an immaculate and tasteful home.

Shep had just gotten out of the shower and Milo introduced him as the "cleanest gang member that ever was." I didn't quite know what to make of this introduction until Milo directed my attention to Shep's impeccable white sneakers and sox and elaborated on the fact that Shep had seven pairs of sneakers because he washes them as soon as he takes them off and they take a long time to dry.

Shep quickly entered a TV trance while Milo and I discussed his latest suspension from school and decision to quit the gang because of a personality conflict with his formerly close friend, Hector. Then Milo asked if I had the camera with me—which I did—and delightedly began viewing everyone through the telephoto lens, making them larger than life-size.

Shep disengaged himself from the TV to share this experience and talked of the opportunity he had in sixth grade to make a film of the decay of his block and to show it to the police and other local authorities in order to precipitate a successful block clean-up. Then he spoke of his reasons for quitting the gang (he had had one ear open all along): too much responsibility—he preferred to do his own thing and let other people do theirs and "the other members were too dirty." I watched this already once-powerful and still highly-respected young man who now rarely entered the world outside of his apartment —inactivity in front of a TV was his way of controlling the helpless anger he felt at the filth outside his door—and watched his animation grow as he held the camera in his hands. You could see that film to him was perhaps the only safe way and complete way of communicating his rage at the dirt and deprivation his people live in. I thought of all the other films waiting to be made—I myself had to turn down requests to me because the center's budget allows only one roll of film a week and it is committed to the street gang project which is very important. But this is not right for people who feel so helplessly unmotivated to be denied a creative act that would make them feel otherwise.

I became involved filmically with the gang at the request of Hector. Hector is president of the junior edition of this division, less than fifteen years old. His older brother is a former president and founder of the entire division and their other brother, Trini, is the current War Counselor. When I first met Hector, I was involved with my photography group and wasn't interested in taking on another group. I have only so much time to give away and prefer to keep my attention concentrated. At fourteen years of age, Hector has got to be one of the world's most sophisticated manipulators. Always keeping peripherally in touch with me, when my photography group terminated he was right there with his project waiting.

Some of the gang's fantasies of me were: 1. a teacher from Hector's school (all of the gang's members are drop-outs and I suspect this was as negative a thing to them as it was to me); 2. a spy on the gang; and 3. a movie star (Trini). These theories are listed in chronological order as my character tests by the gang were met. In all problems of basic mistrust, I feel a consistent presence is the surest cure.

Hector was as defensive of me during this period as I would tolerate. He had had six months to assess and learn to trust me and was impatient for his gang to respond likewise. Now that his negative transference has begun, I look back with nostalgia to this time . . . I say this jokingly because in reality I consider the working through of negative transference as essential to a good therapy as the experience of positive transference.

Tiny (a misnomer) was the president of the gang when we began our film. He was an ideal father figure—macho and dashing, yet respectful, kind, and helpful. He was also discreet with his power and control and interested in helping everyone to do his own thing. He quickly tuned into what I was doing with film and procured a pro-jector and screen for the club. He led cleaning and decorating of the club via a chart delegating responsibility so that there was always some improvement to compliment the gang on when I came. Because Tiny's and my goals and techniques were complementary, I was able to realize my ideal therapy for these boys—a therapy team of a male and a female.

I have no ethical qualms about stating that Tiny was just as good a therapist, probably even better, as I was for these young men. I just think that it's too bad that a good education is contingent upon the ability to procure money instead of the ability to be a therapist. For financial reasons, Tiny had to quit the street gang and is working as a runner for a lone shark.

Drugs

Many times I have been asked my position on drugs with the kids I work with. My feelings on the drugs themselves are similar to those expressed by Dr. Andrew Weil in his book *The Natural Mind* (8). I refuse to be backed into a blanket statement on the use of drugs. I relate to an individual's reasons for drug use. Is he saying,

> "I feel impotent, so look at what a macho daredevil I am for taking this hit of LSD."

"I can't tolerate this painful loneliness and isolation any longer so I will make myself numb."

"I am so empty, I must do this to feel myself."

"I am so depressed, I am immobile; I can't function as others do normally without a hit of speed."

I would no sooner prompt an individual to stop using drugs without getting at his reasons, than I would treat a chancre and think I had cured syphilis. To me, drug use is a defense like any other—in fact, a much easier defense than most for me as a therapist to deal with for the following reasons:
1. Each drug has a distinct "personality." This makes an individual's motivation and feelings about himself easier to discern from his favorite drug selection.
2. Drugs are not a defense accepted by our society. Often a great deal of guilt accompanies drug use, prompting an individual to seek help.
3. Usually, when a person uses drugs, he knows he is indulging in a flight from reality. This makes him an easier person to reach than, say, a religious fanatic.

Under most circumstances, I feel that anyone who has been a drug user and is working with drug users and who does not let his experience be known is wasting a natural resource . . . because at first drugs really do work and users tend to think of nonusers as mentally defective for not getting onto this stuff that can make you feel good. After all, drugs are the American way: "Have a headache? Take Compoz," and "Things go better with Coke."

Some insight can come from talking to a reasonable and together ex-drug user with whom a rapport has been established and who is willing to share his experiences and rationale for change. Unfortunately, there are no magic words or cures that I know of to end drug use.

Sex

A lot of sexual anxiety arose in my seventh- and eighth-grade art groups. As I mentioned, they received no sex education. Also, to make hitting a girl the most awful thing a boy can do (1) sets up many a girl for a kick by a boy who is looking for some awful thing to do with a shitload of displaced anger, and (2) leads the young men to all sorts of violent fantasies about sex ("I heard that if you have sex with a fly* girl she comes out a mess").

I thought it was appropriate to respond to their implied questions and brought in booklets from Planned Parenthood. Milagros had begun to act in a sexually suggestive way with the group which is what aroused the group's anxiety. I wish I could think of a more creative solution, but the rules I have had to set up are that they can draw anything they want but that their behavior must be controlled or the offenders will have to leave. That is my ultimate weapon and I hate to have to use it, but some things are cured only by time and the experience that comes with it.

Summary

From these fieldwork experiences, I've learned the necessity of being receptive to the varying conditions the client sets up for a therapeutic relationship—"different strokes for different folks" so to speak. One must follow to where a client takes you, to experience the world as he sees it—sometimes literally, as with Hector. Simultaneously, the therapist must be careful to maintain the personal distances which are needed to remain objective and which the client needs to feel independent.

A difficult task I think I've mastered is to put my intuition before an authority's advice.

I am still working on my own reluctance to be related to as a woman/mother and on my feelings of responsibility and omnipotence —not really being sure where my responsibilities begin and end, such as with Milagros, or how to handle the subsequent feelings of help-lessness.

---

* "fly" is slang for "good looking."

COMMENTARY

As one reads Barbara's report, imagos appear out of nowhere and give the reader a deep unconscious connection to her field experience. To Heidi, she is both the Little Orphan Annie and the Daddy Warbucks in the dynamic combination of her innocence, her tiny voice and body, and her common sense and straightforward handling of practical and difficult situations. To me, she is the jungle virgin-queen who walks into dangerous situations where others would fear to tread and commands respect and adoration.

There is a libidinal sense that one detects in this entire report. One becomes immediately aware of a raw primitive aggression and sexuality that is tenuously harnessed by the mores of the pack. Barbara becomes much more in touch with the forbidden sexual feelings that seem to be dormant but that are directed towards her, and she is able to handle them with a sense of dignity and graciousness. She helps her men to get a beginning sense of a new conception of women. They do not necessarily have to be kept as possessions and cloistered from a dangerous outside world. The outside women are not necessarily whores who are soiled and exploited. Perhaps they may be a new integration of the tender caring person and the sexual woman. In the gang's mind, however, there is still this division that stems from their shadowy oedipal past. If a woman is sexual, then she cannot be respected, for this means she can be had by everyone. All too often boys in this environment are struggling to emerge from a too close and too sexual connection with their mothers, and they must necessarily compartmentalize their world in order to have some sense of cohesion.

The use of film is of particular import in working with street gangs. The tool can be mastered fairly quickly; there are tangible results, sometimes very gratifying ones. Though there are frustrations in gaining some degree of technical competence, they are not so overwhelming as to cause a despairing withdrawal from involvement. Therapeutically, the gang members have a chance to see themselves in action. And indeed, since they are so close to the border of acting-out, the film gives them a chance to act out not only in safety, but with a pleasure that brings socially-approved results. The gang then has a chance to see these actions and to evaluate what they really are saying about themselves and their lives.

Barbara understands the wide range of complexities that are involved in her work. She visits families and gets a very real picture of what her "sons" must live with. With the guile and agility of someone who knows her jungle, she attempts to manipulate the institutions to work for her rather than to continually undermine any sense of continuity. Thus, she gets the school to keep these adolescents under her supervision even though there are already plans for their transfer. Art therapy in this context must have a very broad base. The therapist must understand what society has done to these teenagers before there can be any work on individual dynamics.

Barbara is no fool when it comes to drugs. She recognizes that if she were to take a moralistic stand with these young men, she would be seen as absurd or foolish. Of importance is that she sees drugs as a defense against real communication and relatedness. Real growth needs and motivations must be fostered before any defense of this nature can really be removed.

The therapist who is frightened of violence will find this a very difficult assignment—perhaps one in which it is impossible to be effective. What remains crucial here is to face one's own fears of loss of control and not to act out by triggering the group either covertly or overtly. Thus, the therapist must avoid power fights and have a very strong definition of self. There must be an openness and acceptance of people and non-moralistic approach. Barbara presents the very essence of this approach, and, as a result, gives the reader some sense of what her secret is all about.

As I write this review of Barbara's work, I think of her intensity and complete involvement in her role as a therapist. Technically, some may complain that she displays over-identification with her men. And, indeed, she has problems in separation and autonomy. Fortunately, these problems work to her advantage as these gangs require a person who is very committed to this kind of work. Art therapy with street gangs demands a very special kind of person. The description of Barbara's work gives us an excellent standard for future art therapists who might venture in this direction.

References

1. Bettelheim, B. *Truants From Life*. Glencoe, Ill.: Free Press, 1955.
2. Bettelheim, B. *Symbolic Wounds*. Glencoe, Ill.: Free Press, 1954.

3. Bettelheim, B. *Puberty Rites and the Envious Male*. New York: Collier, 1962.
4. Searles, H. *The Non-Human Environment*. New York: International Universities Press, 1960.
5. Hansberry, L. *To Be Young, Gifted and Black*. Englewood Cliffs, N.J.: Prentice-Hall, 1969.
6. Allport, G. *The Nature of Prejudice*. Garden City, New York: Doubleday, 1958.
7. Burroughs, W. *Naked Lunch*. New York: Grove Press, 1959.
8. Weil, A. *The Natural Mind*. Boston: Houghton Mifflin, 1972.

14. Art Therapy with a Pre-Symbiotic Adolescent

Linda Joan Brown

INTRODUCTION

The description which Linda gives of her relationship with this handicapped young woman could very well be that of learning to dance with a new partner. There is the same initial frustration with mismatched rhythms, the mutual stepping on each other's toes, and the nonverbal awareness of ongoing messages. But there is also the exhilaration and flow which develop as they begin to move with each other, and the stunning synthesis of developed technique and spontaneous feelings.

Handicapped emotionally far more than physically, Linda's client appears to be profoundly restricted and impoverished. Considering the apparent potential for progress at first, I can imagine that it would be quite difficult not to become discouraged, depressed, or frustrated —reactions which Joanne has undoubtedly met in others many times. The relationship raises many questions, but the most urgent for the student-therapist may be, how does Linda make the transition in their relationship?

It seems that an answer to that question might be that, being well-grounded in experience and psychotherapeutic theory, Linda is able to drop her preconceptions for more natural development. As with smoothly-executed dance steps, this is not so easy as it appears. Recognizing that expectations and fantasies of the kind of patient she wanted are forcing them both into uncomfortable and resistant positions, Linda begins to tune herself to Joanne's actual being and to notice many messages given if only one knows how to look. As she does so, Joanne begins to open to her. In this, Linda illustrates one of the most important qualities that we can acquire in training—the ability to let be. The rewards which Linda describes, the joy in touching Joanne and helping her to respond to another person, seem even to exceed her original expectations.

What appeals to me in Linda's report is her smooth integration of different techniques. Using analytic understanding and a modified form of free association, a "game" by which Joanne returns to her childhood, Linda assesses the primitive level of her client's needs. Then she actively relates to those needs with sensory-awareness techniques and play. She uses art with Joanne to graphically build body concept. Through this and more, Linda unfolds a rich relationship from an originally disappointing encounter—a metamorphosis which could only have occurred through a balance of sophisticated understanding and spontaneous empathy. I find it fascinating to observe in action the flexible and intuitive use of objective knowledge which Linda displays in this case.

THE CASE—JOANNE

I have been working with Joanne for an hour a week for seven months. After four months of art therapy, she was discharged from the hospital after seven months as an inpatient; now she participates as an outpatient in the clinical, educational, and recreational activities of the adolescent program where I work as an art therapist.

Patient's History

Joanne is a 17-year-old black girl who has been treated since birth for cerebral palsy. She is not spastic and retains the potential for normal movement throughout her torso. The CP is mainly manifested in her walk which is characterized by a pronounced limp. She walks without braces.

The hospital records indicate that she had an acute psychotic break with auditory and visual hallucinations, and that upon admission to the hospital she showed "delusions of reference and control . . . verbalizing threatening paranoid ideation." Her visual hallucinations are described as revolving around Moses, God, and the devil, who wore black clothes and had red eyes. God would tell her not to eat and would call her names . . . People stared at her from her bathtub.

Little is known about the precipitating causes of her illness. Possible factors in her history include her having been "dropped" by a boy whom she had been dating in high school around the same time that a female cousin departed from home, and a trauma experienced five months prior to her hospitalization when she was hit by a car and suffered minor leg injury and a blow to the head.

Little is known about Joanne's family history as of this date. Hospital records are incomplete and only minimal contact has been established with Joanne's family. What information is available, through records, family contact and Joanne herself, indicates that, except for the period of her hospitalization, Joanne has been residing with her 80-year-old maternal grandmother since her infancy. Joanne refers to her grandmother as "mommy." Joanne's mother, a diabetic, died of a heart seizure when Joanne was five years old. During Joanne's infancy and early years, the mother lived in a separate apartment with Joanne's father and two older children from a previous marriage.

Joanne was looked after in the grandmother's home, primarily by the grandmother, by cousins and by her half-siblings. The mother, who worked days, would occasionally visit Joanne in the grandmother's apartment on weekday evenings, and she would take Joanne home to live with her on weekends. After her mother's death, Joanne rarely saw her father; she has told me that she sees him, on the average, a couple of times a year.

Included in the hospital records are conflicting reports concerning retardation. Some reports state that Joanne has a history of retardation; others state that she shows no retardation but describe her as having low-average intelligence. Prior to her hospitalization, she was a junior in high school enrolled in a commercial course. Reports from the learning center at the hospital where she is now enrolled indicate that her reading and math skills are at the seventh-grade level.

Some Problems with Countertransference

From the outset of my work with Joanne, I was aware of the difference in our rhythms—my own quick, direct, somewhat impatient gestures and Joanne's sluggish heavy pace. Initially I felt somewhat intimidated by Joanne's remoteness and sullenness. Her intensely closed and rigidly defended manner made me feel hesitant and tentative about intruding into her world. The message I felt emanating from her was: "Get away from me!" When we walked together I tried to slow my step to match hers and found it difficult to tolerate and to sustain. I tried to minimize what appeared to be the threatening effect of my presence by matching her rhythm and using a mirroring technique in the art work. Because of certain unresolved issues of my own, however, I slowed myself down to the extent that I became acutely self-conscious about the slightest movement or gesture I would make. I grew afraid to move, and as time went on, I became increasingly angry and frustrated by feeling so restricted and inhibited, so shut out and pushed out of her world. Through my own wish for merger and my denial of my own separateness, as well as hers, I had turned myself into a non-person.

Slowly I began to assert myself, defensively and defiantly at first: "I refuse to be a non-person." As I introduced more structure into our sessions, I found myself growing pushy and impatient as Joanne persisted in her sparse monosyllabic replies to my questions—and as she retreated from what seemed to be the miniscule advances we sometimes made together in our sessions. Occasionally we would seem to establish closer contact, and at the next session she would come in as defended and closed as before. It seemed as if I had to start all over again each time. I became discouraged and depressed and grew passive. One day in frustration I decided to try and "treat the resistance" and I stated that she was pushing me away. Her response ("You think I'm stupid!?") indicated that she had picked up the accusation in my tone. As I got in touch with my anger after this session—how far short Joanne was of my expectations and my fantasy of the kind of patient I wanted to work with—I began to see my own massive denial of her. Joanne was not the bright, middle-class, verbal, intellectual patient I desired. At this point in her development, she was nonverbal, slow, sluggish and dull. Therapy would be long and painfully slow.

Accepting these feelings—in a sense, seeing Joanne for the first time—brought about an important change in my feelings for her and for our relationship. I found myself more able to relax during our sessions, and, at times, I felt very warm and protective towards her. My observation of her behavior sharpened as I watched for the slightest shifts in movement and expression as signs of changes in feeling and mood. I even began to watch Joanne's hairstyles as possible clues to her feelings at the beginning of our sessions. When her hair was pulled up severely into a knot or into a vertical braid (which reminded me of an Indian warrior), she seemed inclined to be more remote and defensive; when her hair was combed more loosely, she seemed happier and able to talk more freely.

As we continued to work and I began to connect with my own feelings and fantasies about her childhood experiences—of feeling isolated and stigmatized because of her handicap—sometimes I would feel overwhelmed with sadness and the wish to make total reparation for her pain. At other times our growing closeness and Joanne's increased willingness to share herself with me made me feel timid and doubtful of my own ability to handle what I fantasized would be a sudden unleashing of rage and grief as she began to experience her feelings about her disability. Lately, I have also felt burdened and resentful at times with the requirements of the work—helping Joanne means dealing with my own feelings of crippledness. Even as I write this I find myself painfully struggling with them—experiencing something of a "wanting to and not being able to," a helplessness and a paralysis, and, underneath somewhere, glimpses of humiliation, frustration, rage and self-hate. I know that I must deal with my own experience of "I can't" before I can help her deal with hers, and it is becoming more urgent that I do so as Joanne continues to open up. In recent sessions we have talked at length about her surgical operations and about her childhood. We have been warm and close and sometimes it has been difficult for both of us to separate at the end of our sessions. She leans on me as we walk, shares with me the details of her daily routine—her involvement with food, her childlike fantasies of quick and agile trapeze artists and other circus performers. I see clearly her wish to be taken care of, for mothering—and her denial of her limitations, her longing to be the opposite of who she is. Joanne may be more ready than I to deal with these feelings, for I am still working on facing these feelings in myself and on gaining the courage to reflect back to her what she is expressing.

Technical Aspects: Use of Art

Of the materials I made available (cray pas, pressed-crayons, different sizes of drawing paper, water colors, and pencils), Joanne consistently chose to work with the more controlled materials: pencil, pressed-crayons, 9×12 paper. During our early sessions, she would use the straight-edges of the crayon boxes as rulers to guide the straight lines she drew to subdivide the page into geometric shapes. During the first several weeks of our work together, I used the art as a nonverbal method of establishing contact. Joanne's remoteness, her closed and somewhat sullen manner and her reluctant monosyllabic replies discouraged my efforts at establishing a relationship by verbal means.

Mirroring: I began to draw replicas of her designs—imitating the composition and form, line quality, color selections, and the rhythm and pace with which she drew. I did this for a number of reasons— among them, to try and experience the feeling tone of what she was doing and to let her know that I accepted her productions (and therefore her) and found them valuable. Occasionally I would vary my choice of colors, selecting a lighter or darker hue than those she selected; and sometimes I varied the rhythm of my drawing, to see if she would pick up my rhythm and color changes so that we could begin a dialogue through art. From time to time, she did pick up my rhythm; at other times, she seemed stubbornly resistant to acknowledging my presence in any way. During these early sessions, she took her drawings with her.

Soon Joanne began to share the crayons she was using with me, asking if I wished to use the colors she had just finished using. I commented on the difference between drawing fast and drawing slow . . . She said drawing fast was "happier" and that drawing slow was "lazy." This comment seemed to confirm my impression that the slow pace and style with which she drew were partially a defense—that just as Joanne very slowly and carefully colored in the spaces formed by her geometric designs, she was also filling in the time she was obligated to spend with me, without revealing anything of herself to me or involving herself with me in the process. Her concern with reinforcing the lines that formed her geometric patterns, the weak intensity of her colors, the look of emptiness to the page, her somewhat compulsive drawing style, as well as her color choices, hinted to me of her need for structure and control, her lack of ego strength and ego boundaries, her depression and feelings of deprivation, and her ambivalence toward me.

Associating to the Drawings: At the beginning of our fourth session, I decided to stop the mirroring technique and introduce more structure into our sessions. I asked Joanne to draw me a person. She quickly agreed, then changed her mind, saying, "I can't draw . . . I don't know how." Despite my assurances and encouragement, she refused to try. Instead, she immediately began a design, using loose flowing lines instead of her usual geometric subdivisions of the page. When she finished, I asked her to tell me about these drawings, what images she saw in them. She spoke of certain letters of the alphabet . . . "a flying ghost in the sky . . . a sunny day . . . railroad tracks . . . sliding ponds in the park . . . a slinky toy and . . . when you do math with triangles and squares and round circles—a math design." I was surprised by the contrast between the light childlike quality of the fantasies she had produced and her overtly depressed, heavy, burdened demeanor.

At the end of this session, I asked her to sign her name to her drawings, add the session date, and to number them in the order in which she drew them . . . I wanted her to begin to acknowledge her work in our sessions as well as in our relationship; I wanted to start verbally communicating with her about her work. She readily signed, dated, and numbered her drawings, and, for the first time, she left them with me.

At the following session, Joanne spontaneously produced two drawings in which a small stick-figure stood alone in space. The drawings were chaotic and showed Joanne's feelings of helplessness in an overwhelming world she didn't understand and couldn't control. She drew these pictures in an extremely compulsive manner, writing her name several times on each drawing and obliterating her signature with x-s, a star-like symbol—a sign of the anger she turned in against herself and her fear of revealing herself to me.

During the next sessions, we continued to play the "word game" and I wrote down her imagery as she dictated it to me. Frequently her sparse associations had to do with playgrounds and childhood street games (hopscotch, the "lodi game") in which the rules of the game often involved staying within the lines. We talked a little about the wish to control and to make things perfect; as we continued to work and her productions became more figurative so that it was possible for me to see the infantile level of her drawing, I began to relate her need for structure and control to the retardation factor mentioned in her record—a fact I had originally dismissed. I have since concluded, after twenty sessions with Joanne, that her retardation is probably not organic as much as it is a result of emotional factors connected with her and her family's manner of coping with her handicap—factors which have reinforced her infantile dependency needs and her withdrawal from social contact and which have minimized her opportunities for environmental learning.

In the seventh session, in addition to Joanne's usual associations about playgrounds and active street games such as hopscotch, she introduced still another image that related to her disability: "breaks in the knee in different-color pants . . . they need repair." It was time to begin to deal with the issue of Joanne's disability, perhaps using the topic of the playground and childhood games as an opening. At the next session, she again mentioned the hopscotch game. Our discussion went as follows:

    L: "Did you go to the playground with your mommy when you were little?"
    J: "Yes."
    L: "Besides hopscotch, what else was in the playground?"
    J: "Monkey bars, the turtle, and the lodi game . . ."

L: "Were there also swings and a sliding pond?"

J: "They weren't at that playground, but I've seen them at other playgrounds, like the playground near my house."

L: "What was it like for you at that playground when you were small?"

J: "Okay . . ."

L "Did you play with the other children?"

J: "I played with my friends."

L: "It must have been difficult for you . . ."

J: (Silence. . . . I sensed her attention sharpen.)

L: (At this point, I shared with her my own experiences on a playground when I was a child at a time when I didn't know anyone and had no friends—how lonely and sad I'd felt watching the others play, not being part of it.)

"Did you ever feel that way?"

J: "No . . . it was okay . . . I played with my friends."

L: "And your mother . . . did she stay and watch? . . . Was she worried about you and concerned that you be careful?"

J: "No."

L: "Then your mother let you be free to play . . ."

J: (Silence . . . a waiting)

When it came time to end the session, Joanne did not wish to leave and found several reasons to delay her departure. As she left, she asked me for candy, and at subsequent sessions I made certain that sweets were available for her.

Squiggles: At the next session, Joanne asked, for the first time, with pleasure in her voice, "What are we going to do today?" It was then that I introduced the squiggle game. It seemed that by having addressed myself to some of the feelings connected with Joanne's disability, I was finally "in the picture" for her.

From that point onward, the quality of the contact between Joanne and me became more interactive and personal. We did squiggles together and made up drawings together. With evident delight, she helped me paint a table for the new art room where we would continue our work together. Joanne began to greet me by taking my hand and would offer me candy that she sometimes brought to our sessions. She began to talk more freely, and she would occasionally say, "I like coming here."

Clay: After three months, I began to re-evaluate my goals in working with Joanne. Our relationship was established and it was time to formulate a specific direction for our work together. To the 14th session, I brought some play-dough, and as we worked together on building a figure, it became immediately clear how tremendously distorted was Joanne's body-image. She seemed to have no conception of "what comes after the head." She would roll the clay into round balls and then become confused as to how to put them together. At this session I decided that working on body-image was a primary goal —that through building clay figures, I could provide Joanne with a basic learning experience, and that this might be an avenue through which we could begin to deal more directly with Joanne's feelings about her handicap. Since that time, we have built a number of figures in plasticine. All but one of the figures are female (her choice), and she has given them names and ages and made them into a family.

The first figure was that of a woman (see Figure 14.1, Color Illustration, p II). For each part of the body, I asked her to touch and feel herself and to look in the mirror "to see what's there." She would then look at me as I touched myself in different places. We began with the head and named the parts as we went along. Through this process, Joanne's sexual blocking (hinted at in her earlier drawings) became strikingly apparent. I added a breast to the figure we were building and asked her to add the other. She added a piece of clay and very carefully proceeded to flatten it down. She "forgot" the pelvis and was wondering how to add the legs to the chest. For the legs, she rolled the clay into a ball and placed it under the pelvis we had made. This reminded me of the stick-figure she had drawn in our seventh session where the female figure had only one leg, perhaps signifying Joanne's "good leg." I showed Joanne how to divide the sphere into two parts and roll the clay into legs. She still uses this procedure to make the limbs. The sphere for Joanne seems to be a primary symbol, perhaps representing breasts and nurturance as well as her preoccupation with childhood games. It is also reminiscent of the art work of very young children, in which the limbs are drawn as emanating from the head.

For six sessions, I continued to do mirror-work with Joanne— encouraging her to see and touch the different parts of her body, to feel and compare which parts were smaller and larger, and to notice how the different parts of her body connected and moved. I also began to incorporate my skills in sensory awareness into our work. For a while, we would begin each session with breathing and movement

before proceeding to our work with clay. Working with our bodies—
with breathing and touching one another—helped promote an increased closeness between us.

After the first two sessions with clay (in which we built the figures
together and Joanne then traced on paper and colored in the figures
we'd made), she began doing most of the clay work on her own. The
figures grew progressively smaller until she made a figure of a baby
girl protected by a blanket in a crib (see Figure 14.2, Color Illustration,
p. H). As she was building the figure of the baby, we had the following
discussion:

> L: "Do you remember when you were a baby?"
> J: "Yes . . . four months before I was born . . ."
> L: "What was it like?"
> J: "Sleeping a lot and eating food and kicking . . ."
> (At this point, the sequence, as I remember it, is unclear. The
> fantasy seemed to change from the inside of the womb to outside,
> and I'm unclear as to whether this change occurred through Joanne
> or through me. We continued, talking about the sounds that babies
> make.)
> J: "Babies say 'Daddy,' 'Mommy,' 'milk,' 'food,' 'soda' . . ."
> (She was talking with obvious enjoyment about this.)
> L: "It seems that that was a happy time for you."
> J: "Yes."
> L: "Sometimes I think it was happier to be a baby than to be
> grown up."
> J: "I know what you mean . . ."

In this session (and through the progression from adult-figures to
child-figures), Joanne seemed to be saying on one level that she could
not deal with being a grown-up woman (with sexuality or being independent and taking care of herself in the world) and that she saw
herself as a baby or would find it more comfortable to be a baby. Her
fantasy about the womb indicated confusion and perhaps curiosity
about women's bodies and where babies come from; perhaps it reflected some wish to have a baby. At the same time, her enjoyment of
our breathing exercises and movement, which addressed themselves
to her adult body, indicated to me that we must work simultaneously
on both the child and adult levels.

Since this session, through the creation of stories about the figures and drawings she has produced, I have continued to explore Joanne's fantasies as well as the reality of her childhood, we have talked at length about her leg operations during her childhood, and she has acknowledged some of the fear she experienced in this regard. I am slowly learning more about her family history and how she presently spends her time at home. As the opportunities present themselves, I may begin working with Joanne on sitting, standing and walking activities which will necessitate even more of an acknowledgment on her part of her feelings about her handicap. Gradually, I may want to get Joanne onto the floor (paper body-tracings or a childhood game like "jacks" might be vehicles for doing this)—for it is on the floor that the sensory awareness work becomes most effective in unblocking breathing, becoming aware of body boundaries, getting acquainted with the idea of the floor and ground as support, and, through the use of guided imagery, awakening and using the senses and becoming aware of the sensations and energy requirements of small and gross movements.

However, while the sensory work has both educative and therapeutic value, I view it as only one of a number of possible directions that my work with Joanne may take. Joanne is beginning to take the lead in our sessions (e.g., suggesting during our last session that we go outside for our meetings), and working with whatever feelings Joanne expresses during our meetings remains the primary goal.

COMMENTARY

Linda's case highlights a number of important aspects pertaining to the treatment of severe depression. This patient's development is fixed at a early stage. Indeed, as we observe the tremendous degree of impoverishment and lack of self, one might guess that this patient's problem is essentially a pre-symbiotic one. In other words, the very early connection between mother and child was so poorly defined and worked out that we have a patient who is virtually enshrouded in a sense of deadness and isolation. Other depressives are much nearer the level of separation and individualization. Thus, the patient has made enough of a closure with the maternal source, but gets caught up in an introjective battle because of the fear surrounding separation and abandonment. In the case that Linda is presenting, there is very little introject to speak of.

As Linda attempts to mirror and become related symbiotically to this patient, she recognizes her sense of futility in feeling or being fused with her. To be true, she must face her own feelings of disappointment in working with a patient who is of dull-normal intelligence. However, as the therapist starts to take hold of the case and to structure and direct it, something seems to happen. The patient responds in a very positive and affirmative sense. Thus, the long path of mothering and feeding this patient—along with a whole wealth of stimulation and imagery—has begun. This is the curative process of such a case. Sensory awareness, dance therapy, guided fantasy-play, the sharing of the therapist's own imagery—these are all excellent techniques for nurturing this patient's growth.

Linda is wise enough not to start on a verbal level with this patient. If in no other area, the art therapist brings a very special resource to the treatment of a case like this. This patient's ego resources and verbal tools are so poorly developed and ill-defined that to engage in a therapeutic dialogue on the verbal level is too difficult a burden. As patient and therapist enter into the nonverbal realm, they truly make contact with one another.

Linda is able to recognize when art is used as a resistance. All too often art therapists receive meaningless designs from their patients and do not see their underlying meaning: These works are often strictly an evasion from any really meaningful communication. Linda breaks this pattern and redirects the flow of communication. If one does not take an active stand with this kind of patient, one can get lost in a state of nothingness.

Linda understands the profound importance of body-identity in this case. Indeed, this is an issue which reappears in several other reports, such as that of Ellen's work with her youngster. But in contrast to Ellen's child, this patient's sensitivity has been deadened from a lack of stimulation. Seemingly, sensitivity techniques were made for this patient. And those techniques that can be directly hooked up to a body-awareness are particularly useful.

Art therapists come upon this problem of barrenness and emptiness in any number of settings. The subsequent drain on personal resources is immense since they must literally pour themselves into these patients. When this massive investment does occur, the results are usually quite favorable. A common fear among beginning therapists who work with these patients is one of either infantilizing them or feeding their dependency. In cases where this is really an issue, the therapist discovers that giving only serves to foster regression. This is not the case with Linda's patient. She responds beautifully to Linda's encouragement and interest and neither misuses nor basically exploits the relationship.

The beauty of this case seems to lie in Linda's realization of the real needs of her patient and in her ability to give to one human being who is embedded in a very deep sense of nothingness. The dedication that she expresses will be required of others who venture to work with patients who have suffered similar deprivations.

15. Art and Nonverbal Experiences with College Students

Susan E. Gonick-Barris

INTRODUCTION

Susan's work with education students in a college setting represents a humanistic dimension in art therapy—the premises that we experience a basic need to create and that the arts hold dynamic potential in facilitating self-actualization. Another element, highlighted by her choice of placement, is the responsibility she takes for affecting the quality of education, an issue which concerns her deeply. Susan's sense of purpose and commitment to her techniques refreshes and excites me—especially as I remember the floundering which some of us experienced at first, and the calming effect of learning with someone who believed so deeply in what she was doing. It occurs to me that this deep self-commitment must be an essential quality in successful therapy. I know that it attracted me to her immediately as a resource of thoughts and ideas.

As her fieldwork account illustrates, Susan's spirit is highly contagious. I still cannot determine whether her magic comes from natural charisma or carefully cultivated skills—probably both. She actively exercises her ability to play, to laugh at herself; yet at the same time she can take herself and others very seriously when necessary. She displays a straightforward ability to demand and to get what she wants; consequently, she can encourage and inspire others to do the same. She is willing to feed people when she can and to admit when she can't, after which she almost always is able to suggest where you might find what you were looking for.

Perhaps one of the reasons she seems so at home in her work is that she has carefully chosen her professional territory. She takes on what she can handle comfortably. In these student groups, Susan offers experiences to which she herself responds. In fact, she offers a wealth of actual techniques to increase sensory awareness, to relax constricted bodies and minds, and to start creative sources flowing. Her willingness to share and to develop new material with all of us seemed to keep me in touch with what it is like to be going through these experiences for the first time.

Susan's fieldwork report is permeated with the genuine freshness and involvement which she maintains in her sessions. Surely much of her vitality and commitment originates in her background as an artist. It seems appropriate that an artist would be the one to introduce us to forgotten selves and to make lost senses come alive.

THE CASE—COLLEGE STUDENTS

My fieldwork project was to give a series of workshops for students at a state college. The workshops were to offer experiences in group art —using arts and crafts media as tools for personal growth, exploration of interpersonal relationships, and examination of fears and resistances which blocked the free-flow of creativity. Members would explore a variety of materials and experiment together by communicating through color, shape, line, form and texture. In this paper I will describe the workshops I gave and the experiences we all shared.

After sounding out several friends who were graduate students at the college as to which instructor would be most receptive to something innovative, yet consistent with the course goals, I was referred to Dr. Taylor in the education department. An appointment was made and I found her to be a gracious and independent spirit. I left some information with her about my background as an artist and educator.

The following week I met with her class to discuss the workshop with them and to set up a schedule for those students who wished to participate. Dr. Taylor offered her class members the choice to participate or not, as they each wished, and she gave me an opportunity to respond to their questions. I was surprised at the many fears expressed of "not being good enough in art" to do anything. Most students needed a good deal of assurance that an art background was unimportant and, in fact, that sometimes "art training" could be a handicap. I stressed the "play" aspect of the experience and emphasized that nothing would be judged, evaluated, or "produced." As I left, Dr. Taylor told me that she would telephone me that evening if there were sufficient interest in what I had offered. To my delight, she called that evening to let me know that eight students had volunteered and would meet with me for two hours on the next Tuesday.

When I met with the group I was prepared to do several different kinds of things but decided to wait until I could sense what the group flavor was. I started with the statement that in this workshop we would try to experience ourselves, using the art materials as an extension of feelings. I explained that each individual was free to withdraw from the activities if uncomfortable, that each should take responsibility for participating or not.

The first ten or 15 minutes of the workshop was spent "focusing on internal states" with eyes closed. I had learned this in one of my theater classes and had found it to be an excellent warm-up and preparatory experience. Much sensory-input is often below awareness; therefore I asked for a deliberate focus on pressure, temperature, sensations, feel of feet on the floor or back against a chair, clothing, etc. After standing up, we tapped our heads with the tips of our fingers, experienced the space between limbs, changed space by moving, and finally opened our eyes to make nonverbal contact with a partner. Each couple was given a large sheet of white paper and some oil-pastels. They were asked to look at one another and then mutually to decide—without words—who would start and who would follow. My directions were to begin drawing—without once lifting the crayon off the page—anything to which their eyes were attracted in their partners' faces. They could each return to whatever was most interesting but should be sure to keep the line continuous. As each partner finished, the other was to have a turn; when both were finished, they were to talk together about what they saw on the page. (With some modification, this is a classic drawing experience developed by Kimon Nicolaides as described in his book *The Natural Way to Draw*. Nicolaides was not interested in technique; he was dedicated to finding and releasing the creative impulse of each student. He believed the essence of an art experience was the emotional connection between the artist and his subject.)

After this first exercise, I asked the students to change partners. We continued doing this until each had had several partners and several different line drawings. The subsequent group exchange, after we pinned all the pictures up on the wall, dealt with how surprising and new these familiar faces had become. Aspects of faces were discovered that had gone unnoticed. There was much humor and very little self-consciousness since the drawings were very abstracted and no likenesses were expected or attempted.

Large lumps of clay were then distributed to each person. I spent a few moments talking about clay: "This is plasticine. It is hard and will require your body heat and energy to soften it. Please do not 'program' your clay. Let it be what it wants to be. Do not try to make a model of anything with it. Work with it. When you are finished, place the piece on this table. Place it to reflect where you would feel most comfortable if the clay were *you*. Near the center? The outside? Near someone you know? Or someone you would like to know better?"

As they started to work, I played a record which I had brought along. The music was a beautiful flute concerto and slowly people seemed to relax with the clay and really get into the material. Some sat with legs folded; some stretched out on their stomachs; some lay on their backs holding the clay in the air. Everyone was very absorbed (me too). When our time was almost up, I asked for the clay to be placed on the table.

This part of the workshop could have gone on for hours. Everyone had a great deal to say about their "position" and about how they arrived at their final "shape." There were long monologues of shape-to-image-to-association-to-previous-experiences . . . of memories long-forgotten and poignant statements from several people. The clay became the skeleton key to a hundred different rooms. Near the end I suggested that those who wished to change the position of their clay, do so. Half of the group felt moved to do just that. Our time was up and we couldn't believe that two hours had come and gone. Everyone wanted to come back and was disappointed that two hours was all the time we had. (In order for everyone to have a chance at the workshop, no one was allowed to come twice. I was given three weeks—after which everyone in Dr. Taylor's class was to begin student-teaching assignments and would no longer be in her class.)

That evening Dr. Taylor called to tell me that her class had heard from this group; the report was that they were "ecstatic." Their experience sparked a good deal of interest in those who had been undecided and the rest of the class now wanted to come to the next workshop. We set a date for the following week. I limited the group size to ten members—because I believe a smaller group has a more intimate feel and works better.

The next week, eight students appeared for the workshop. They seemed much looser and my approach was a little different: We started by getting acquainted on the blackboard. My instructions were "Draw something on the board about yourself relating to your mood: Choose chalk in a color or colors which express your mood. Use anything that will communicate that mood to us—a symbol, a shape, a line—to tell us where you're at. Shapes can be large or small, anything that expresses how you feel in any way which might connect the rest of us to you." I began first; each person took a turn in no special order. Everyone chose to participate, and, when each had taken a turn, I asked who would like to talk about the chalk-work. No one did, so I went first again. I talked about my nervousness and about what the colors of my lines meant to me. I was honest and brief. After my turn, everyone took turns without hesitating. This experience—which I had intended as an ice-breaker and was using as an introductory experience, expecting it to last only about ten minutes—seemed to have created something very special within the group and no one wanted to leave it until an hour had passed. In response to my Pratt group's asking for a sample of my work, I repeated this experience with them. There was the same intense participation and wish to continue; in fact, we spent two class sessions with it.

I wish I had had the presence of mind to have photographed the students' mural because nothing I can say with words could adequately express the surprising quality and the remarkable beauty of it. The group was unusually expressive and we spent an hour on this part. The blackboard was about fifteen-feet long and was covered with large brilliantly-colored sections in assorted shapes, symbols, and lines. After we discussed our "piece," I asked if anyone wished to change or add in any way to the whole. Some people did. From a distance, the board looked like an exquisite Persian rug. Some sorrow was expressed that we couldn't take it or copies of it with us somehow. Little signs were tacked around it saying "PLEASE DO NOT ERASE US." Reluctantly we disengaged ourselves from the chalkboard and made peace with the fact that we couldn't "hold on" to it.

The next experience was a nonverbal dialogue with oil pastels. My instructions were for each person to choose a sheet of paper from a large stack of multicolored papers. Then each was to choose a partner nonverbally, and the couple was to sit on the floor with the paper between them. I asked them to try to relax and look at each other. They were to know their first impressions. One was to start first, putting something on the paper—a thought or feeling without pictures. All expressions were to be abstract. Only one of the papers was to be used, and both partners were to take turns alternately. After about ten minutes I asked the couples to turn the pages over. The other side was to be more specific—each partner was to express something about the past or a truly significant event. I told them to use symbols and to create their own symbols, too. If it were really important, they could use a word but not more than one for any one turn. I had planned to allow about ten minutes for this, but the group pressed for more time. After about twenty-five minutes I had to end this part. I asked the couples then to exchange explanations with each other on what they had drawn or written. What happened on one side? What happened on the other side? I asked them to take turns pinning up their paper for a group-sharing of the material (if they wished). A great range of emotion was expressed. Many appeared very surprised at this. Everyone was eager to talk and to share significant life events (not all of which were heavy, by the way; some were humorous). People seemed at ease and comfortable with whatever was talked about.

After a while someone said, "This feels like group therapy . . . is it?" Other comments were "I feel as though a cork has popped and I can pour . . ."; "You know, now I'm feeling a little bit sad . . ."; "I wish we could stay all morning . . ."; "I've thought of things I hadn't thought of for years . . ."; "Are there places I can go where I can do more of this over a long period of time?" "Could my boyfriend and I go to one?" "Do you give these things privately? Can I come?" "I feel very warm towards everyone here, and when we return to the class, you people will be more special to me . . ." When they left, they thanked me and expressed the hope that I would return. I noticed a real difference in the expressions on their faces . . . even in the way they moved. They seemed brighter-eyed and more animated to me. I remember two things very clearly: One was a sense of exhilaration for having facilitated such a meaningful and pleasurable experience, and the other was a wish to have acquired magically a videotape of the event. People will think I am exaggerating, I thought. I wanted proof—that their eyes did shine and their mouths were unscrewed, that their gestures were smoother and their walk more flowing.

On my way home, I experienced a great let-down and began to dwell on the enormous responsibility of "opening" people. I started to become a bit depressed at the thought and then wondered whether my little "success" was now going to fuel some unexpected self-defeating behavior.

A few days later I spoke with Dr. Taylor again; once more she gave me some delicious feedback. The students expressed such delight with their experience that she herself would like to participate. We set up another (and final) workshop for the following week. She also told me that some students had wanted to come again for a second turn, but she had to turn them down until everyone else had had a first chance.

The next workshop was the smallest—with only four students instead of the ten expected. I couldn't help but wonder whether it was chance or Dr. Taylor's presence. Although she was a very friendly and direct person—and did not send out any authoritarian messages—I couldn't help but think her presence had in some way accounted for the lower attendance. Actually I was affected by the fact that she was there. I know she had come in good faith—out of an earnest desire to taste a new dish—yet I could not relax enough to be my own "me" in the easy and informal style that had characterized previous workshops. Instead I dwelled on the quite absurd notion that she was there to judge and evaluate me. No one knows better than I do that nothing good can flower in such a climate of distrust. However, in this small group of five we did the previously described chalkboard statements and the "significant event" dialogue on paper.

In spite of my nervousness, things went well; people seemed to enjoy the event and were open enough to say that at first they had hoped that Dr. Taylor would not show up (I was unable to admit this). We talked together about the value of these experiences, and there was unanimous opinion that art is an important and under-used way to foster communication. One student said, "This is a great way of seeing yourself or presenting yourself to others, rather than by looking or speaking . . ." Someone else said, "This is a good way to find a common relation with others through 'drawn' experiences and feelings." Dr. Taylor's comment was that although she did not gain any personal insight, she learned about others and thought it was a very good experience. She, too, would have liked more nonverbal experiences. Another student said he enjoyed the workshop because he was not a verbal person; he had discovered that he could reveal more of himself through art as other people do in verbal conversations. He said he was usually very uncomfortable talking with others—even those people he knew—but this time it was easy, and he had not experienced the usual handicap.

COMMENTARY

Drama, movement, music, and art are woven into a Gestalt that renders art therapy dynamic, alive, and exemplary of the tradition of creativity and humanism. Susan's perception of art therapy is setting a direction for the future growth of this field. Art therapy cannot be limited to the use of visual tools to enhance creative and therapeutic growth. To limit its boundaries is to violate the very essence of artistic expression. The expressive fields need to be integrated, and Susan demonstrates how this can be done.

She weaves in sensory awareness techniques and psychodrama; she borrows from dance movement. She speaks as an artist who is very much involved in creation and will not pay lip service to artificial boundaries or so-called professional roles. She asks her students to flow with the material; she requests that they likewise let the material flow into them.

A number of cogent issues are raised by Susan's report. Of deep concern to Susan—as well as to the entire field of mental health—is one of using these workshops in a manner that will neither do harm to nor cause disruption in the transient participant. As Susan is rightfully concerned, she does not want to open up vulnerable areas in her participants and then leave them hanging. Her technique is a demonstration-workshop and, by its very nature and goal, must be limited. The workshop leader must be very aware of the power of this tool and must be able to use it subtly, carefully and lovingly. One hears all too many accounts of workshop participants who have been overwhelmed by material that has broken through their defenses. Thus, the workshop leader must be trained in sensing limits as well as bringing about closure. The leader must also be sensitive in picking up the signs of desperate people who may occasionally filter into these workshops and who present a very disruptive influence. There are also people who have developed a style of communication, acquired from attending other workshop programs; that can make it an unauthentic and sterile affair. In other words, they have picked up the lingo of the human potential movement. Susan is very much aware of these issues and handles her role with a good deal of integrity and responsibility.

Another problem which seems all too common in Gestalt techniques is the sterile application of role-playing or dramatic exercises.

Spontaneity and creativity of the art therapist are diminished with the repetitious use of such techniques as "What does the color say?" or "Have a dialogue between your right and left hand." A Gestalt approach in its truest sense must take into account all the field forces that are accruing and then creatively weave them into a here-and-now situation. In other words, the art therapist's technique must come out of an organic sense of the situation. The same criticism can be directed toward psychoanalytic approach which focuses on the past as a way of giving rational explanations rather than really helping the person experience important phenomena in a very dynamic sense.

The polarization of various approaches in this field seems to be counter-productive as well as antithetical to the creative growth experience. To integrate the Gestalt here-and-now approach with a multiplicity of expressive modalities and to couple it with a depth approach to the unconscious and to ego defenses are goals that would seem very appropriate to the field of art therapy.

Susan's concern is, in part, with the field of education. With her characteristic initiative and maturity, she attempts to bring about change in a typical undergraduate program. This is pioneering work. Someday in the future, there will be many more workshops and courses of this kind so that education will be directed towards the whole person.

III. APPLICATIONS

16. Art Materials

This is your first professional job. The staff and administration are enthusiastic about you but know very little about art therapy. You are given a bare room and a limited budget, and are requested to implement your program. What kinds of supplies do you buy? Strictly art? Craft kits? Educational toys? How do your materials express your approach to creativity development? What emotional responses are inherent in a particular material? Perhaps some of the ideas presented in this chapter will help to answer these questions.

All too often art therapists restrict themselves to one or two basic materials. Different media, however, provoke different kinds of messages. Some address themselves to the ego-organizing capacity of the patient. Other materials tap very deep libidinal levels, while still others have an exploratory quality. Some challenge a sense of mastery; others provide just pure fun. Hopefully, an art therapist can work towards becoming an expert in the broad use of materials which supply the needed communicative links in everyday therapeutic situations.

Although we realize patients often have their choice of all available materials in an art room, their creative experience is ultimately the responsibility of the therapist. Sometimes she may simply guide the patient's choices, while at other times she may present a specific activity. She may also offer a choice of materials that represents opposite qualities, allowing the patient to communicate his needs.

Materials can emphasize the various polarities of a patient's intrapsychic life. A patient who is drawn to hard, aggressive materials, for instance, may need a gradual introduction to round and soft experiences; armature wire can be molded into soft curvilinear shapes or made into sharp, spikey aggressive projections. A doll house can offer a cozy enclosed space. Patients benefit from exposure to these opposites; they need to experience help with materials, to let go as well as contain them—to be able to push in and insert as well as to receive. By highlighting and bringing together polarities, materials add richness to an individual's experience.

The art therapist must assess the stimulus potential of a medium as well as the ability of her patient to cope with and integrate excitation. For example, finger paint makes high demands on a patient's ability to control and manipulate fluidity, rhythm and texture. This can be too much of a challenge for an acting-out patient. On the other hand, a tightly restricted or depressed patient might find some release with this material as it opens the gates for a needed regression. Thus, the quantity, textures, malleability, and chromatic stimulation of materials are all parts of the assessment of stimulus impact.

First, however, the art therapist should look at the patient and the particular developmental stage requiring attention. Is the need for comfort, organization, or mastery? Is regression a factor or does he need broadening and reflections of his inner life? Does the patient need, and can he tolerate, a challenge in the form of a new material? Will the material be too threatening to the adult self or, on the other hand, will it be a road to a thwarted infantile impulse?

Since the art therapist works, for the most part, with groups rather than individual patients, she should also be able to transpose some of these principles within a group dynamic approach. The group then is assessed as a unit and responded to in terms of its capacity to handle stimulation.

Touch and texture are important dimensions to consider in assessing a particular medium. Some materials have a soft quality, while others feel harsh or brittle, and a few are sticky, tight or tough. The art therapist who is truly resonant with her patient may be able to introduce material that corresponds appropriately to the patient's needs. Some patients have a void in the area of touch and sensorium while others, threatened by too close contact, need a slow and gradual introduction to texture stimulation. For example, a lonely removed child may slowly work his way from paper dolls to tempera, watercolor to clay, and finally to soft textured materials as parts of a collage. Involved in this kind of progression is an opportunity to begin with distance and control, gradually increasing exposure to stimulation and psychomotor release.

Jung (1) states *colors* may be attributed to the four functions of perception and judgment: green for sensation, yellow for intuition, red for feeling, and blue, thinking. Luscher (2) also developed a well-known color theory. The art therapist may play with some of these notions and hypothesize an intrapsychic map based on the patient's reliance or avoidance of certain colors. She may also give the patient the freedom to choose colors that express his current emotional state as well as set in motion a dialogue in contrasts and alternations. The individual who denies blackness and dysphoria with excessive use of white spaces may need a breakthrough via dark or chromatic materials. Likewise, a preoccupation with dark heavy affects may need exposure to the vitality of yellow and orange. The cold rationality of blues may require the spontaneous childlike expressions of pinks or reds.

The color inherent in any particular material has its expressive as well as defensive qualities that need appropriate responses and remedies (3). The therapist who assesses the energy locked into the color of a material can offer an additional experience that either harmonizes or contrasts with the crosscurrents flowing from the patient. Color is more often a consideration when using two dimensional materials, i.e., paper and paint, markers or crayons. But think of the stimulus impact of terracotta clay as contrasted to white porcelain clay; the former is more basic and primitive, while the latter seems more controlled and pristine.

Specific media may also be broken down into various components. Clay has a range of textures and stimulation: rough and abrasive; wet and gushy; elastic and short. Ball clay will stretch and twist, while plasticine is tighter and holds its molded shape better. Play dough offers smell and color as added ingredients for stimulation and direction but lacks the permanency of plasticine. Paper also is a common material with a multitude of tactile messages. Think of the difference in feeling quality among the following papers: colored construction, foil, oak tag, corrugated, tissue, velour, kraft, magazine, newspaper, lace, wrapping and notebook. Amazing! Even white drawing paper and manila each have a distinct touch characteristic.

Materials also have their particular characteristics in terms of *movement and rhythm.* Some media are easily controllable while others demand a connection between an inner and outer flow. Some media can be avoided in the early stages of a treatment relationship as they demand too much flexibility and freedom of movement. The patient who is struggling with mastery and dominance may find stone an excellent testing ground to explore these conflicts. Stone requires strength and a force of precision but does not always respond predictably to pressure and must be respected for its own internal harmony and movement. Watercolor demands a willingness to be spontaneous; oil offers a more predetermined and exacting challenge. The latter takes weeks to set and dry and likewise demands a test of one's patience. Woodcarving has some of the same rhythm requirements as

stone and gives a clearer roadmap for a patient to follow because of the
texture and movement of its grain. Clay, on the other hand, can be
pushed and shoved in a multitude of directions and can offer a wider
range of possible expressions. Metalwork dances and moves as it becomes hot and fluid. With the bubble and flow of hot metal there
is a tremendous sense of excitement as something very basic and
powerful starts to emerge. Armature wire helps the patient push and
pull and express conflicting tensions or, if there is a loss of control, he
may end up in a tangled mess. Another example of contrasting
rhythms is linoleum printing versus potato printing. The former entails a controlled but aggressive movement and includes more extensive planning and execution. The latter results in a repetitive
motion and gives quick, easy results. Thus, the determination of the
most appropriate task includes an evaluation of the age and coping
capacity of the patient.

Space is another component quality of a particular material. Some
media have their own boundaries; others are flexible. Some activities
are enclosed, as in a sandbox where the patient can feel safe and avoid
the fears of a swallowing environment. The antithesis might be Elaine
Rapp's technique in which music, tissue paper and movement are
involved, and the patient is required to throw, catch, hit and swirl (4).
As body, material and movement intertwine, feeling free and comfortable with movement in space is a necessity. Plaster may be experienced as inviting, threatening or releasing. A metamorphosis may
happen before one's eyes as the wet amorphous flow becomes hard
and brittle. Plaster also changes from warm to cold in temperature.
Clay moves from soft to hard but takes days to accomplish this
transition. The environment, objectified and contained through
murals done on large expanses of paper, also requires body movement.

Movement in space implies different requirements on one's mus-
culature. A contrast might be between crocheting, weaving, and
making jewelry as opposed to hammering, chopping or welding. Some
people have a large rough body movement orientation while others
prefer small precise movements. Some patients need encouragement
in dealing with more freedom in movement; others require material
to contain their impulses and to bind energy. Certain materials have
their own inherent structure, while others offer a wider range of
choices and possibilities. One example of this dimension can be
found in working with hospitalized children, who often experience

their environment as manipulative and chaotic, with an accompanying loss of control. These feelings can be counteracted by building with materials that have a structural quality, such as popsicle sticks, building blocks, Lincoln Logs or Tinker Toys. The child constructs a part of his own world and feels a sense of mastery. The repetitive safe quality of the activity is a way of dealing with the pervasive confusion and overwhelming change in his life. Children who have come to terms with the hospital experience can then move on to handle the more expressive experience of clay or paint. The transition from a safe repetitive structure to the more fluid changing material can be molded and remolded to fit a changing understanding of the environment.

Changing our perspective, we can consider the *concrete or abstract qualities* of materials. Some media have prescribed courses or structures to follow; others demand a continual flow of abstractions and probably have a more expressive quality associated with them. It is important to recognize those patients who need something concrete and specific, where a crafts orientation provides a comfortable meeting ground between therapist and patient. The geriatric population offers a case in point. Often this group needs something tangible that produces concrete results. At times, older persons present a rigidification of thought processes and a diminution in their ability for abstraction and expression. They may feel threatened by a request to paint or draw and may need a stimulus such as a poem or story to ignite images. Georgiana Jungels (5) has satified this need by collecting antiques, everyday objects common during the beginning of our century. When shared with a group of older people, these objects stimulate memories, dreams and images which act as connecting links between past and present and among group members.

Risk-taking varies from material to material. Some patients, frightened of mistakes or errors, soon learn to capitalize on accidents as a rich new avenue for expression. The patient may learn this through stone as he increases his capacity to change adversity into victory. Any subtractive process, such as working with wax, soap or wood, demands taking risks. Once the patient removes or separates a material, there is no moving back. Clay, on the other hand, tolerates mistakes because the process is additive as well as subtractive. Thus, the concepts of reversibility, decision-making and flexibility are inherent qualities of an activity.

Working with art materials can provide a microcosm of the real world. For instance, the setting-up of an inner world can be dramatized through sandbox play, giving a patient the opportunity to recognize intrapsychic processes (6). It can also act as a practice field for the changing and manipulation of interpersonal relationships. The selective use of materials then leads to trial and error behavior and offers an opportunity for new alternatives in the future.

Patients may choose materials that restrict horizons rather than encourage therapeutic communication. The practitioner must be constantly on the alert to assess the resistance value of a particular material, i.e., stereotyped or repetitive communications. The range of materials used by patients and the security value that arises from a constant reliance on one medium are other aspects of this problem.

Different media offer a range of opportunities for stimulating feelings of *mastery and competence*. For instance, the tissue paper collage is a sure success: It is abstract, only requiring the patient to glue one torn shape onto another and the brilliant color combinations ensure a visually appealing result. By contrast, the use of oils entails considerable skill and control. It is all too easy to end up with a mess. Patients whose abilities are limited by skill or patience should stay away from this medium. In many instances, the introduction of an easily mastered activity at the beginning of a relationship may give the patient the needed confidence to take greater challenges in the future.

Some materials more readily lend themselves to *fantasy play*. Miniature figures of people, animals and villages can stimulate dramatic play on a mural, clay base or road map and help the therapist and patient clarify important life themes. Other patients, particularly children, need to use material to express ill-defined symbols. Body-tracing with markers and large mural paper can start the process of building a symbol of the physical self. Dolls, puppets and masks can express through dramatization various part-images and introjects. Cardboard boxes and construction paper often help to concretize the outside world when used, for example, to make spaceships, trains, doll houses or play country stores. With these representations, a child has the opportunity to take a fantasy journey through play and discover the various conflictual energies contained in his inner life.

Many individuals need an opportunity to conceptualize and contain a shattering and split-off world. The Polaroid camera gives a live reflection of this world and at the same time gives distance, space and containment to the experience. The camera works as a synthesizer as well as an observing ego. The immediacy of the picture captures the reality and makes it possible to digest in small parts what previously seemed overwhelming. In psychological terms, the ego has an opportunity through this medium to become increasingly differentiated and autonomous. Movies and video have some of the same attributes and offer the added opportunity of capturing a series of movements in a more realistic, alive fashion. To play back and study behavior that has been dissociated and repressed can make an important therapeutic contribution.

Junk sculpture is an excellent means for helping a child evaluate and value his world, to let him know that things that seem lost may be rediscovered and once again become useful. Some patients who have been discarded by the family or society need to experience this lesson. This sculpture expresses a particular kind of mastery: What others consider junk not only has value but provides an avenue for expressing a newfound creative identity.

As we review the subject of materials, the range of considerations posed by each seems overwhelming. Ideally, familiarity through use will allow the therapist to be aware of touch, color, movement, rhythm, risk, and space considerations, as well as symbolic content. This information will be integrated with clinical and environmental demands so the therapist may offer the most appropriate activity or choice of activities.

Media can be used to build or uncover; they also connect, as well as express, outer and inner life experiences.

Art therapists often rely on intuition as to the use of an appropriate medium. The conceptual and cognitive understanding of a psychology of materials will strengthen their ability to make a therapeutic impact. This knowledge of materials and the subtle and creative use of media to facilitate process differentiates them from psychotherapists who occasionally utilize art materials to enhance therapeutic communication. From this vantage point, materials are very organic to theory, technique, and the practice of creativity development and therapeutic change.

References

1. Jung, C. G. *The Archetypes and the Collective Unconscious.* Translated R. F. C. Hull. Princeton: Princeton University Press, 1959. p. 355.
2. Scott, I. A. Editor and Translator. *The Luscher Color Test.* New York: Random House, 1969.

3. Birren, F. *Color Psychology and Color Therapy: A Factual Study of the Influence of Color on Human Life*. New York: McGraw-Hill, 1950.
4. See Chapter 17, Techniques. Function: Building Out, Focus: Mastery of Materials, #1.
5. Jungels, G. Presentation, American Art Therapy Association Convention, New York, 1974.
6. Kalff, D. M. *Sandplay*. San Francisco: Browser Press, 1971.

APPENDIX A
MATERIALS

Paint
tempera
oil
acrylic
water color
finger paint
food coloring
enamel
india ink

Clay
ball clay
plasticine
terracotta
porcelain
play dough
carran d'ache
bread dough

Printing
linoleum
silkscreen
batik
potato
vegetable
sponge

Sculpture
plaster
wax
soap
wood
wire
metal
junk

Handwork
knitting
crochet
macrame
applique
quilting
doll making
needlepoint

Crafts
leather
popsicle sticks
ceramic tiles
models
plexiglas
beading

Papers
drawing
manila
construction
canvas board
tissue
corrugated
foil
oak tag
cardboard
sandpaper
newspaper
velour
wax
paper towels

Utensils
crayon
pencil
magic markers
charcoal
ink pen
cray pas
pastels
conte
brushes
sponge
Rich Art markers
Flair pens
palette knife
X-acto knife

Adhesives
Elmer's glue
rubber cement
contact cement
epoxy

Other
sandbox
Polaroid
videotape
super-8 movie camera
35 mm slide camera
tape recorder
typewriter

17. Technique

"What is art therapy?" "What do you do?" "How do you do that?" "What skills and techniques are involved?" We have all been asked these questions and all felt uncomfortable or somehow unable to answer them satisfactorily. At times, as practicing art therapists, we have all reached for a technique either to help a patient towards a therapeutic goal, to relieve our own anxiety, or both. While we have dealt with the specific problems of theoretical and professional definitions elsewhere, here we would like to offer a catalogue of techniques presented within a theoretical framework relevant to the therapeutic relationship.

To begin defining "art therapy technique," let us separate the component words of the term. *Art* speaks of originality, individuality, a creative process; graphic materials, colors, textures; spontaneity, risk, alternatives and imagination. *Therapy* implies taking care of, waiting, listening, healing, moving towards wholeness, growth-provoking, medicine, human exchange, sympathetic and empathetic understanding. *Technique* connotes structure, rationality, mechanical, unfeeling, industrial, calculating; a skill acquired by repetition and familiarity. The meanings of the individual words combine and rest on a sound theoretical base of psychotherapy and creativity to constellate our definition. The individual definitions seem to cancel each other out. Perhaps it explains why art therapists in the past have encountered difficulty in communicating exactly how they practice. Nevertheless, there is little question that students and professionals need to have a framework that can be tested, communicated and shared as an orderly basis for future growth (1, 2, 3, 4).

An art therapy technique is a concrete implementation of theory introduced by the art therapist, at the appropriate time, to facilitate creative and therapeutic change. While there is some overlap, techniques can serve three separate purposes:

Projective techniques are more often used for diagnosis of the patient; *research techniques* are employed to gather objective information; *therapeutic techniques* are used to enhance communication in the therapeutic session. The last category most concerns us here.

Some patients need very little in terms of technique from the art therapist. They are self-motivated, self-actualizing people, who, when given the proper atmosphere, interact with the therapist. At times, this atmosphere is referred to as technique. We prefer, however, to relegate the atmosphere to the axiomatic givens that should be a part of *any* educational, therapeutic and growth situation: the respect and regard for the individual worth of the patient; a definite contract for uninterrupted space and time; the establishment of care and trust in the relationship; the presence of a therapist who is emotionally available and connected to her patient, and who has the capacity for an empathetic relatedness that is neither identified with nor too distant from the patient.

For many others, however, the process of creative self-development needs much more. The process gets stuck and bogged down. There is a deadening, vapid aura that surrounds the interchange; the art work becomes sterile and repetitious. Somewhere the patient is frightened of moving forward and retreats into a welter of defenses. He may be frightened of letting go, opening up or just daring to take a peek at some of what is going on inside of himself through an expressive act. The mere presence of available materials and a good trusting relationship is not always enough. The questions then arise: How do we move? How do we begin the dialogue? At this point the therapist may make a creative statement to the patient to break through and reach the patient's hidden self. This creative communication cannot be contrived but must be discovered and extended with a dynamic sense of aliveness and authenticity. This communication is what we call technique: It recognizes the patient's fear of growing as well as his opposing wish to change. It is our understanding of how to respond to these forces that will jar the energy balance and result in a release of self-actualizing material.

To a point the collected material reveals where we are as a profession regarding art therapy technique. Towards self-development, we often adapt psychotherapeutic techniques; towards creative growth we often adapt art education techniques. The survey that follows includes techniques developed also from happy accidents, as well as creative solutions to therapeutic problems. Many of the art projects presented were not new or extraordinary. Their appropriate utilization and

underlying rationale make them useful and exciting. The specifics of
implementation—why, how, when and what—are all too often determined by chance or solely by the intuition of the therapist. This
chapter is in no way meant to be a gourmet guide of recipes intended
to remedy that situation. To simply extract an idea (i.e., puppets because you just watched "Sesame Street"), without making the related
considerations, is not only anti-therapeutic, but may be destructive.
Technique is only one element of a network of component parts com-
prising the therapeutic situation. This can be no substitute for a
sensitivity to the specific patient population, relevant issues, goals,
atmosphere and setting.

In essence, cognitive understanding must accompany feelings and
intuitions for effective implication. All of the above factors contribute
to the therapist's response to a patient via an art therapy technique
that will facilitate the ongoing process. We realize this task requires
years of education, practice in the field and, most of all, continuing
personal growth on the part of the therapist.

Information for this survey comes from four main sources:

(1) Personal interviews conducted at the 1973 convention of the American Art Therapy Association in Columbus Ohio;
(2) A questionnaire distributed to students in the Pratt Institute Graduate Art Therapy Program;
(3) Telephone interviews with members of the New York Art Therapy
Association;
(4) Perusal of the complete works of the *Bulletin of Art Therapy* (5)
and the *American Journal of Art Therapy* (6).

The questions used in personal interviews can be found in Appendix
A, and the questionnaire given to Pratt Institute Graduate Art Therapy
students can be found in Appendix B.

There is no attempt in this chapter to include all techniques. We
do, however, hope to give the reader a way of understanding and
integrating the existing material.

The collected information from interviews and written responses
has been correlated and presented within the following format:

Technique: the title or descriptive name of the activity.

Materials: the kinds of preparation and things needed before starting a therapy session.

Directions: how to use the materials; how the script may unfold.

Population: age and general physical or psychic condition of patients technique was used with and may be adapted for.

Issues: probable and possible topics raised as a result of introducing this technique.

Therapist: the specific individual who contributed this concept. Often, ideas were reported by several therapists. Where possible, the original source has been indicated. Inclusion of the therapist's name will hopefully give credit where due for originality, but does not imply exclusive use or patent rights. Often, therapists shared experiences and feelings that would make these sparse descriptions come alive. Unfortunately, the way the collection grew and developed does not allow for a prose description of individual applications. Most therapists listed here are members of the American Art Therapy Association. On their behalf we extend an invitation to contact them should you desire further information. To all contributing students and therapists we offer our sincere appreciation for sharing their experiences. We hope they have been interpreted accurately and that others are aware enough to adapt these specific implementations to their own needs.

The techniques are divided into three large categories according to their *function*: Toward what goal does the therapist aim to use the energy released through the activity? The term *focus* indicates the specific area of development the technique intends to facilitate. Depending on the particular individual or patient group, the current life problems being experienced and/or under discussion, the therapist may wish to focus awareness through the introduction of one of these techniques. Further explanations of individual areas precede the groupings of techniques. It is hoped that the original poems preceding each focus will communicate a sense of the patient's subjective feeling experience.

The first function category we have called *Building Out*—from the core of a person's identity; communication and perceptual skills; understanding self in a relationship to others, etc. The second function category may developmentally follow the first—*Revealing and Discovering* the self. How is energy used to bring together existing parts of the self and understand them further? An awareness of the inner world is emphasized here. *Integrating* techniques comprise the third function category. Here energy is used to pull together the inner and outer worlds of the personality in an attempt at further individuation. Adequately understood and creatively employed, some techniques can be used for all three functions. We are less concerned with a doctrinaire system than with providing material for innovation and application.

BUILDING OUT

Building Out translates as structuring and constructing the patient's image of himself in relation to the world around him. While image and ideation come first, in this area the therapist also helps the patient experience, comprehend and integrate his interpersonal interactions within his environment. Developmentally, art therapists may originally find themselves focusing on an awareness of the patient's sense perception, body schema, visual-motor activity and cognitive skills. If one is to explore the outside world, a point of reference is essential. This group is labeled *Me, The Patient*.

Me

Who am I? My self, my voice, my body, my name. This feeling of me, not you. Uniquely me-in-this-world, in my room alone. How do I see, hear, touch, feel? What's my history? herstory? Where have I come from? been? going? My dreams. I am learning to do—I can't do this but I can do that. My freedoms and limitations. Stretching myself always to make me, me!

FUNCTION:	*Building Out*	*FOCUS:*	*Me, the Patient*
Technique:	Paste Up Autobiography.		#1
Materials:	Paper, old magazines, glue, scissors.		
Directions:	Find images from magazines and photographs that represent your life.		
Population:	Adolescent; adult.		
Issues:	Reinforcing my physical reality.		
Therapist:	James Denny (7).		
Technique:	Shoebox Camera.		#2
Materials:	Shoebox, scissors, markers.		
Directions:	Cut a hole in the box for a lens and take imaginary pictures. What is significant in this room? Objects? People?		

Population: Adolescent; adult; neurotic.
Issues: Focus on what I find meaningful in the environment.
Therapist: Elaine Rapp.

Technique: Simon Says.   #3
Materials: A wide open space to move.
Directions: Children follow the leader game; change leaders.
Population: Children up to 8 years.
Issues: Building body awareness.
Therapist: David Tavin.

Technique: Felt Board.   #4
Materials: Masonite board, felt background, scissors, cut-out felt,
                  figures, letters, house, window, car, face with features, etc.
Directions: Use in conjunction with crayons and paper, written word
                  and touching relevant part of body or toy or thing.
Population: Child, autistic.
Issues: Perceptual training, spelling, patterning
Therapist: Pam Glick.

Technique: Stringboard.   #5
Materials: Homosote board, hammer, nails, colored string or thread.
Directions: Draw a circular pattern in pencil, hammer nails on out-
                  line, one inch apart, wind thread around and around to
                  create an image.
Population: Child, autistic.
Issues: Centering; release of tension in hammering, eye-hand
                  coordination, pressure, concepts of around and back and
                  forth.
Therapist: Pam Glick.

Technique: Smells.   #6
Materials: Perfume, spices, soaps, flowers.
Directions: Always combine texture and smell with visual image.
Population: Child, mentally retarded.
Issues: Alternate ways of learning.
Therapist: Rosalind Seldigs.

Technique: Setting the Table, Household Chores.   #7
Materials: Varies.
Directions: Involve parents in therapy by consultation and com-
                  munication of goals; chores can provide practice area.
Population: Child.

FUNCTION: *Building Out*   FOCUS: *Me, the Patient*
Issues: Perceptual training: left/right; top/bottom; sweeping
                 broom towards or away from you.
Therapist: David Tavin.

Technique: Textured Numerals and Alphabet.   #8
Materials: Corrugated cardboard, felt, velvet, burlap.
Directions: Cut out letters and numbers from cardboard with each
                 side a different texture.
Population: Child, dyslexic.
Issues: Recognition of figures, i.e., b and d and p; Z and N.
Therapist: David Tavin.

Stepping beyond the entirely egocentric stage, the therapist will find ways to initiate the therapeutic dialogue. Establishment of a flowing communication between patient and therapist is, of course, necessary for further development of the process. These techniques fall under the heading *Me and One Other*.

Me and One Other

Me and you. Separate. Hard to hide. You care, why? Do I trust? Or run? You are here, intensely *Here* for me. I need no help. I want no help. Can you hear me? Stay away!! Stay, maybe we can share. Do it together, share and trust. Don't talk but share an ocean walk.

FUNCTION: *Building Out*   FOCUS: *Me and One Other*
Technique: Face Painting.   #1
Materials: Acrylic paint, soft brushes.
Directions: Using the face as a canvas, paint an abstract design or
                 expressive mask. Uninterrupted time; one to one.
Population: Child; adolescent; adult.
Issues: How do I see you? How will you paint me? Trust and
                 perception.
Therapist: Janet Adler.

Technique: Sharing the Drawing Space.   #2
Materials: Paper and markers, pencil, crayons or pastels.
Directions: Have a nonverbal dialogue in images; create an environ-
                 ment for the two of us to exist in; exchange color or
                 medium after a while.

Population:	Child; adolescent; adult, withdrawn.
Issues:	Safe means of stimulating involvement; introduction through images.
Therapist:	Joel Barg.

Technique:	Sharing a Constructive Activity, just the two of us. #3
Materials:	None.
Directions:	Yardwork, shopping outside the hospital and then role-playing the activity afterward.
Population:	Adult, psychiatric hospital.
Issues:	Trust, appropriate behavior, comprehension.
Therapist:	Robert Ault.

Technique:	Portrait Impressions of a Partner. #4
Materials:	Paper and crayons or cray pas or markers.
Directions:	Create a portrait of your partner only in colors and shapes, non-figurative.
Population:	Adolescent; adult.
Issues:	Sensory perception.
Therapist:	Linda Brown.

Technique:	Role Reversal: P teaches T a skill. #5
Materials:	Open.
Directions:	Allow P to teach you a craft or skill, i.e. needlework or oragami.
Population:	Child; adolescent; adult.
Issues:	Statement of belief in worth of P; role-playing of authority; I'll only ask you to do what I'm willing to do also.
Therapist:	Jil Lustgarten.

Technique:	Therapist as Secretary. #6
Materials:	Paper and pen, quiet.
Directions:	T takes dictation and types letters, poetry, stories.
Population:	Child; adolescent; adult, particularly geriatrics.
Issues:	Role reversal; respect for thoughts and power of communicating them; teach mail system; encourage contact outside the institution.
Therapist:	Ann Watson, Helen Landgarten.

Technique:	P and T draw and exchange paper to work further. #7
Materials:	Paper and markers or crayons.
Directions:	Draw for specified amount of time, either free or theme oriented.
Population:	Adolescent; adult.

FUNCTION: *Building Out*   FOCUS: *Me and One Other*
Issues: How do I regard your creation? What's the message?
               Differences and similarities in color, mood, tension, etc.
Therapist: Michael Edwards.

Technique: Problem/Solution Diptych.   #8
Materials: Paper and markers.
Directions: Fold paper in half. P and T each draw a problem on the
               left exchange papers, and draw the solution on the right.
Population: Adult, psychiatric.
Issues: Problems solving, reality testing.
Therapist: Shellie David.

Once the relationship gets going, patients may need their world
expanded further; connections must be made. Perceptions of the
family may be vague and diffuse and seem unrelated to the therapeutic
encounter. Incorporation of the self-image and interpersonal environment can be explored and horizons widened through techniques under
the headings of *Me and the Family* and *Me and the Peer Group*.

Me and the Family

Who am I to them? They to me? Sometimes we, then again me.
Separate from them. We/me/they. Love, how? Manipulate and want
to kill, give a kiss, make a present, compete, separate. Parents and
power. A need to be loved, feeling ignored, important for survival and
must outgrow and the constellation changes for a lifetime.

FUNCTION: *Building Out*   FOCUS: *Me and My Family*
Technique: Houseplan.   #1
Materials: Newsprint and crayons.
Directions: T draws house plan and asks P to indicate family mem-
               bers and describe activity.
Population: Child.
Issues: Awareness of roles; relatedness to family; environment.
Therapist: Harriet Cheney.

Technique: Paper Dolls and Animal Zoo.   #2
Materials: Paper, scissors, pen.
Directions: Fold and cut animal families and paper dolls; evolve a
               story with the P as you proceed.

Population:	Child, withdrawn and mentally retarded.
Issues:	Assessment of growth and development; relatedness and feelings about family.
Therapist:	Emery Gondor.

Technique:	Sociogram.	#3
Materials:	Paper and pastels, markers.	
Directions:	Graphically illustrate yourself as the center of a wheel and your family around you; closeness to center indicates importance of tie, time spent with, emotions invested in.	
Population:	Adolescent; adult.	
Issues:	Taking an objective look at interrelatedness of members.	
Therapist:	Elaine Rapp.	

Technique:	Family Tree.	#4
Materials:	Paper and markers.	
Directions:	Make a tree and assign a part to each family member; list age and relationship and feelings towards.	
Population:	Child, where there is no access to records.	
Issues:	Who's left out? Power struggles, favorite parent, etc.	
Therapist:	Linda Beth Sibley.	

Technique:	Family Mobile.	#5
Materials:	Cardboard, coat hanger and string.	
Directions:	Construct a three-dimensional sociogram of family members representational or abstract.	
Population:	Child.	
Issues:	Can child see family as a unit with stable and moving forces?	
Therapist:	Pat Newell-Hall.	

Technique:	Paper Sculpture	#6
Materials:	One piece of construction paper, glue and scissors.	
Directions:	Quickly make something.	
Population:	Family art therapy group.	
Issues:	Individual and family focus, projective technique.	
Therapist:	Helen Landgarten.	

Me and the Peer Group

Equals. Sameness. Difference. Ages alike and worlds apart. Consciousness begins and oh, what pain, partners, groups. A new family—

only different, equal. More freedom and more responsibility. Best friends, yet reluctantly respectful of friend's other friends, possessive, jealous, competitive, devoted, depressed, excited. Teamwork, cooperation; changing insides all the time.

FUNCTION:	*Building Out*	FOCUS:	*Me and Peer Group*

Technique: Cooking a Meal Together.   #1
Materials: Kitchen, food and serving area.
Directions: Plan, shop, prepare, serve and enjoy a meal. Alternate roles if done on a weekly basis, i.e. host, guest and chef.
Population: Adolescent, hospitalized.
Issues: Teamwork, allocation of responsibility, planning, handling money, manners, reading recipes, cleaning up.
Therapist: Leslie Abrams.

Technique: Puppet Show Videotaped.   #2
Materials: Fabric, socks, paper cups, styrofoam, buttons, cardboard, etc., paper plates, yarn.
Directions: Suggest story line analogous to recent experience of group. More directly, act out upsetting occurrence.
Population: Adolescents, hospitalized.
Issues: Feedback, useful for other staff, sublimation and integration.
Therapist: Nancy Bagel.

Technique: Newsletter or Magazine.   #3
Materials: Stories, poems, drawings, cartoons, riddles, puzzles and a printer or Xerox machine.
Directions: Collect, design, print, distribute all contributions from group; ongoing project.
Population: Adolescent; adult.
Issues: Task oriented, ventilation, creativity respected, communication to other staff regarding patient feelings.
Therapist: Joel Barg, Mary Steele.

Technique: Round Robin Drawing.   #4
Materials: Paper and markers, crayons.
Directions: With group sitting in a circle, draw for 1–2 minutes and pass your drawing to the right until it completes the circle.
Population: Adult.
Issues: Group unity, drawings as indicator of group identity.
Therapist: Linda Brown, Julia Housekeeper.

Technique:	Group tied together with string.	#5
Materials:	Several balls of colored string.	
Directions:	Tie yourselves together as a unit; move, dance, get a cup of coffee.	
Population:	Adult.	
Issues:	Cooperation.	
Therapist:	Cliff Joseph's Group Art Therapy class.	

Technique:	Feeling Charades.	#6
Materials:	Paper, pencil and a hat.	
Directions:	Each member writes an expression of feeling on paper and puts it into a hat; feelings acted out in turn for identification.	
Population:	Adults, psychiatric hospital.	
Issues:	Experiencing feeling levels nonverbally.	
Therapist:	Sonia Moscowitz.	

Technique:	Group Sociogram	#7
Materials:	Mural paper on the floor, markers.	
Directions:	Graphically illustrate community relationships.	
Population:	Adolescent; adult, residence.	
Issues:	Interrelationships, decision-making, cooperation.	
Therapist:	Leslie Abrams.	

Technique:	Mime and Drama.	#8
Materials:	Stories, plays.	
Directions:	Choose work analogous to life situation, i.e., *The Lottery* by Shirley Jackson.	
Population:	Adolescents, deaf and mute.	
Issues:	Nonverbal communication, body awareness, comprehending material.	
Therapist:	Linc Reinhart.	

Technique:	Mural with Moveable Cut-Out Figures.	#9
Materials:	Mural paper, drawing paper, scissors, color crayons, pastels or markers, masking tape.	
Directions:	Ask each group member to draw a full figure self-portrait; cut it out and tape it to the mural paper in the place the patient finds most suitable for himself. Each person may change his own placement or others', to best describe how he sees the group. Allow the group to come to a consensus on the final placement of the figures and then create an environment for them on the mural.	

FUNCTION: *Building Out*   FOCUS: *Me and Peer Group*
Population: Adult, psychiatric hospital.
Issues: Group identity, interpersonal relationships, leadership size and placement of figures.
Therapist: Mickie Rosen.

Technique: Theme Mural with Interchangeable Cut-Out   #10
               Figures.
Materials: Mural paper, drawing paper, scissors, color crayons, pastels or markers, masking tape.
Directions: Place cut-out figures on to a group mural depicting a fantasy theme, i.e. "The group has been stranded on a desert island. We've made a life for ourselves, now a rescue ship is in sight, but it does not have room for all (another ship will be along in the future). Who will go? Who will stay?" "We are in school. The teacher is absent and there is a substitute. How will the class behave?" or "We have gone on a picnic. What will we do? What will it be like?"
Population: Adult, psychiatric hospital.
Issues: Separation, frustration, tolerance, cooperation, peer relationships, authority, etc., depending upon the fantasy situation offered by *either* the therapist or the group.
Therapist: Mickie Rosen.

Technique: Solar System.   #11
Materials: Styrofoam, wire, string and paint.
Directions: Three-dimensional sociogram using planets as people.
Population: Child; adolescent, school.
Issues: Interrelatedness from general science interest.
Therapist: Wendy Wulbrandt.

Technique: Wooden Dolls.   #12
Materials: Flat wooden doll family, tree, car, house, 8–10" tall.
Directions: Trace and compose a picture.
Population: Adult, psychotic.
Issues: Reality testing, projection, body awareness.
Therapist: Maxine Whiteman.

Technique: Group Sequential Drawing.   #13
Materials: Large paper and markers.
Directions: Draw and pass to create a story.
Population: Adult, psychiatric hospital.

Issues:	Collective statement of focus.
Therapist:	Shellie David.

Technique:	Silhouette Mural.	#14
Materials:	Mural paper, markers, scissors, slide projector or spotlight.	
Directions:	Silhouette body parts, cut out, arrange on mural.	
Population:	Adolescent.	
Issues:	Introductory group experience, body awareness.	
Therapist:	Cynthia Wolf.	

Technique:	Filmmaking with Street Gangs.	#15
Materials:	Super 8 film equipment.	
Directions:	Film your world, print, edit.	
Population:	Adolescent street gangs.	
Issues:	Identity, respect for equipment, body image.	
Therapist:	Barbara Maciag.	

Technique:	Filming Group Process.	#16
Materials:	Super equipment, masks.	
Directions:	Short film describing activity of growth of the group allegorically in mime and dance.	
Population:	Art therapy students.	
Issues:	Learning equipment, cognition of emotional process integration.	
Therapist:	Cliff Joseph Group Art Therapy.	

As awareness-of-self grows outward and becomes awareness-of-self-within-an-environment, a patient begins to see social and political groupings beyond the level of family and friends. Art provides ways for safely exploring the outside world through practice in fantasy. Increasingly, art therapists see themselves working with patients outside the consulting room or art studio and opening up direct communication with and in the environment.

Me and the Community

Who's in this with me? A hamlet, a town, a city, a country—the global village via TV—*how* many of us *are* there??? What are the rules? Where can I go? How to relate to busdrivers, cashiers, police and teachers? Kids—younger and older than me. Grandparents; dogs and cats; others' property; signs that say No *Trespassing* and *Welcome*! What's a museum? an aquarium? a bodega? a community day? How do you pay? Who does the work? Let's do it together.

FUNCTION:	*Building Out*	FOCUS:	*Me and the Community*
Technique:	Fantasy Community.		#1
Materials:	Mural paper and markers.		
Directions:	Discussion and drawing. Who will we admit? Where shall it be? laws? leaders? recreation? schools? housing?		
Population:	Adult, psychiatric hospital.		
Issues:	Freedom and responsibility in all areas of life.		
Therapist:	Jessie Bighach.		

Technique:	Miniature Village.	#2
Materials:	Cardboard, plaster, papier mâché and construction paper.	
Directions:	Create a three-dimensional town in miniature, changing the appearance to suit occasions and seasons; semi-permanent in the art room.	
Population:	Adults, psychiatric hospital.	
Issues:	Outside life versus inside hospital; awareness of seasons and cyclical processes; vehicle for story-telling.	
Therapist:	Toby Gross.	

Technique:	Take a walk, play basketball, visit a museum.	#3
Materials:	Free time.	
Directions:	Spontaneity in response to need.	
Population:	Adolescent, one to one.	
Issues:	Courage to move from safe therapeutic space and relate to a large environment.	
Therapist:	Leslie Thompson.	

Technique:	Telephone.	#4
Materials:	Old telephone or play phone.	
Directions:	Keep available for use anytime for fantasy conversations.	
Population:	Child; adolescent.	
Issues:	Teaching skill in using; practicing communicating and reaching out.	
Therapist:	Bob Wolf.	

Technique:	Role-playing with Hats.	#5
Materials:	A collection of hats, i.e. police, fire, detective, nurse.	

Directions:	Choose a hat and speak for that person in your town; what does he do, feel, touch, how does he relate?
Population:	Child, schools and hospitals.
Issues:	Awareness of how I and others function in community; what I would like to be or do; why did I choose to be that person?
Therapist:	Linda Beth Sibley.

Technique:	Map-making.	#6
Materials:	Paper and markers.	
Directions:	Draw my bus or walking routes from home to school; school to Scouts, etc.	
Population:	Child, dyslexic.	
Issues:	Patterning, following directions, awareness of environment, left and right.	
Therapist:	David Tavin.	

Technique:	Refrigerator Box Houses.	#7
Materials:	Huge box, paint and mat knife.	
Directions:	Create your own house or several to make a neighborhood.	
Population:	Child.	
Issues:	Personal environmental statement; openings, doors, windows, number of rooms, color, space, etc.	
Therapist:	Ann Watson.	

Technique:	Theme Centered Collage.	#8
Materials:	Magazines, paper, scissors and glue.	
Directions:	T chooses relevant issue and Ps respond by selecting pictures that convey a feeling response in collage form.	
Population:	Adolescent; adult.	
Issues:	Open.	
Therapist:	Susan Mann.	

Technique:	Matchbox Car Mural.	#9
Materials:	Collection of miniature cars and mural paper.	
Directions:	Create a road system, road signs, territory, towns, schools. Detour, yield, slow down. . . . and play!	
Population:	Child.	
Issues:	Response to environment and directions, movement for active kids; stimulus for fantasy.	
Therapist:	Madeline Tisch.	

FUNCTION: *Building Out*   FOCUS: *Me and the Community*
Technique: Ragdolls.   #10
Materials: Old sheets, scissors, thread and needle, pattern, fabric
                 scraps, cotton for stuffing, yarn for hair.
Directions: Cut, sew and stuff happy and sad soft dolls to be used
                 for pre-operative teaching for surgery.
Population: Parents of children in hospital.
Issues: Occupies parents during operative wait, provides kids
                 with a better understanding of procedures.
Therapist: Madeleine Petrillo.

   A patient needs various ego skills to survive and deal with the
world around him. A mastery of materials not only provides the tools
for creative expression but can accurately parallel personality development. Art educators bring special strength to this area including perceptual judgment, patterning, and synthetic and organizational
abilities. Included below you will find materials that stimulate growth
on several levels simultaneously.

Materials

   Look mom! I can build! I can bend and fold and sew and form and
dance. I can make a mess. I can write a story, make a movie, be a
robot, ride a rocket. Look at what I can do! (But I can't draw a
straight line.) Here's a present. It's like magic. Want to learn how?
I'll show you!

FUNCTION: *Building Out*   FOCUS: *Mastery of Materials*
Technique: Tissue Paper Sculpture.   #1
Materials: Colored tissue paper, armature wire, glue and music.
Directions: Pick a color you resonate with, throw, catch, swirl it to
                 the music, move your body freely; then stop and combine
                 the wire and paper to make a sculpture capturing that
                 feeling.
Population: Adolescent; adult, neurotic.
Issues: Integration of sound, space and color movement and
                 feeling.
Therapist: Elaine Rapp.

Technique:	Carpentry.	#2
Materials:	Wood, hammer, nails and saws.	
Directions:	Make an abstract wood sculpture.	
Population:	Child, autistic.	
Issues:	Concrete structured activity that releases tension.	
Therapist:	Pam Glick.	

Technique:	Needlecrafts—Weaving, Needlepoint, Macrame.	#3
Materials:	Loom, yarn, canvas, markers, cord, pins, and scissors.	
Directions:	Individual projects or group with wall hangings; don't ignore boys and men!	
Population:	Adolescent.	
Issues:	Sensory-motor coordination, follow-through, frustration tolerance.	
Therapist:	Olive Galdston.	

Technique:	Scratchboard, and Magic Pictures.	#4
Materials:	Crayons, India ink, stylus, cardboard.	
Directions:	1) Paint a picture with colored inks, cover with black crayon and scratch away a design with stylus; 2) Crayon a picture, paint with black India ink and colors show through.	
Population:	Child; adolescent; adult.	
Issues:	Sure success and neat trick to capture imagintion with combination of materials; concepts of addition and subtraction.	
Therapist:	Deborah Oberfest.	

Technique:	Junk Sculpture.	#5
Materials:	Popsicle sticks, bottle caps, foil, broken game pieces, and glue.	
Directions:	Create a sculpture, mobile, collage with found objects.	
Population:	Adolescent.	
Issues:	Acceptability of non-formal materials for making art; ability of student to make a creative statement of value from others' garbage.	
Therapist:	Leslie Thompson.	

Technique:	Butterfly Painting and Potato Printing.	#6
Materials:	Paper, paint, potatoes.	
Directions:	1) Glop paint on center of page and fold in half; 2) cut potato in half, carve design and dip in paint to print.	

FUNCTION: *Building Out*   FOCUS: *Mastery of Materials*
Population: Child; adult.
Issues: Sure success of these and other art education projects pro-
                 vides atmosphere for development of trust and willing-
                 ness to relate.
Therapist: Randy Faerber.

REVEALING

All of the above techniques have something to do with the building
of the patient and his relations to his outside world. But what of his
inner world? The inside part is composed of lost images, disorganized
and conflicting affects, fantasies and myths. How does the art therapist
relate to this world, particularly when avenues of entry are protected
by road blocks which only serve to further embed and alienate the
patient from himself?

Revealing translates in our terms as conscious discovery of more
unconscious, less obvious aspects of the self—gathering information
and recognizing ways of perceiving. This process is more analytic in
approach than Building Out. Identifying and understanding these
characteristics of being fall into four main areas: *feelings, sensations,
thought* and *intuitions*. These techniques are applicable to patients
who are already functioning on fairly mature levels of integration and
who seek more self-awareness. At times one finds these techniques
demonstrated in workshops or in settings with fairly normal populations, perhaps college students.

The expression of much repressed feeling is a central road to travel
if we want to become aware of unconscious forces affecting our perceptions, judgments and behavior.

Feelings

Am I hot, cold? Comfortable. That's good, no good? Feeling
rejected, accepted, ignored, loving, close, distant, left out. ANGRY,
furious, scared, admired and envied. Hate, passion, stiff and awkward,
very tired, well welcomed, blue, green and yellow success. Where does
it come from—this continual flow of feelings, MY feelings???

FUNCTION: *Revealing*   FOCUS: *Feelings*
Technique: Drawing Emotions.   #1
Materials: Paper and markers or crayons.
Directions: Ps execute quick abstract drawings in response to T's
                spoken word, i.e., love, hate, anger, depression.
Population: Adolescent; adult.
Issues: Identification of emotion in relation to color, shape,
                pressure.
Therapist: Mala Betensky.

Technique: Masks of Affects.   #2
Materials: Papier mâché, paint, found junk and egg cartons.
Directions: Choose an emotion and make a mask that expresses it.
Population: Child; adolescents.
Issues: Follow-through on an important feeling.
Therapist: Janet Adler.

Technique: Clay Monsters.   #3
Materials: Ceramic clay, glaze and kiln.
Directions: Create a three-dimensional monster, fire and glaze, from
                either fantasy or dreams.
Population: Adolescent.
Issues: Concretization and assimilation of scary feelings.
Therapist: Leslie Abrams, Robert Ault.

Technique: Finger Painting to Transactional Analysis Statements. #4
Materials: Finger paint, special paper and a close-by sink.
Directions: T makes child, parent and adult statements, i.e., "Let's
                play," "Go to your room," "I appreciate your opinion."
Population: Adolescent; adult.
Issues: Connection to feeling role states.
Therapist: Elaine Kirson.

Technique: Group Mural.   #5
Materials: Mural paper and pastels.
Directions: Discussion of theme followed by each P's responding by
                individually going to mural and drawing; discussion.
Population: Adult, hospitalized.
Issues: Leadership within group, relevance of theme, connection
                or dissociation from topic.
Therapist: Cliff Joseph.

Technique: Angry People Collage.   #6
Materials: Construction paper, glue and magazines.

FUNCTION: *Revealing*   FOCUS: *Feelings*
Directions: Cut out pictures clearly expressing emotion and paste into a collage; write a dialogue for each character.
Population: Adolescent, adult.
Issues: Ventilation, acceptance and assimilation of strong negative emotion.
Therapist: Helen Landgarten.

Technique: Draw Situation Depicting Feelings.   #7
Materials: Paper and crayons.
Directions: Draw yourself in a stressful, joyful, helpless, controlling, etc. situation.
Population: Adult, hospitalized.
Issues: Observing ego defense mechanisms and/or responses to a specific situation.
Therapist: Myra Levick (7a).

Technique: Draw your Earliest Recollection.   #8
Materials: Paper and markers.
Directions: Draw earliest and next earliest recollection and relate to present situation via discussion.
Population: Adolescent; adult.
Issues: Influential memories, beliefs, continuing themes through life.
Therapist: Susan Mann.

Technique: Draw Your Mother Criticizing You.   #9
Materials: Paper and markers.
Directions: Change family member and action to suit each patient.
Population: Adolescent; adult.
Issues: Observing ego in a feeling interaction.
Therapist: Susan Mann.

Technique: Gesture Drawings.   #10
Materials: Large pad of paper and charcoal.
Directions: Make a gesture that communicates an inner feeling and further articulate gesture into drawing that you find most clear.
Population: Adult.
Issues: Combination of feeling, movement and visual representation; release of energy.
Therapist: Ben Ploger.

Technique:	"I am a window and . . ."	#11
Materials:	Storytelling poster or large blown-up photo.	
Directions:	Select a part of the photo and become it and speak for it.	
Population:	Adolescent; adult.	
Issues:	Gestalt exercise in projection of feeling and identification.	
Therapist:	Elaine Rapp.	

Technique:	Exploring Holiday Symbols.	#12
Materials:	Paper, markers and scissors.	
Directions:	On appropriate seasonal holidays, ask for feeling associations to be drawn and discussed, i.e. hearts, crucifix, flag.	
Population:	Adult, psychiatric hospital.	
Issues:	Personal versus cultural meanings of symbols.	
Therapist:	Bernard Stone.	

Technique:	Feeling Judgments.	#13
Materials:	Paper and pastels.	
Directions:	Draw the person I hate, admire, love, envy the most.	
Population:	Adult, psychiatric hospital.	
Issues:	Awareness of feeling projections; acceptability of a wide range of emotion.	
Therapist:	Bernard Stone.	

Technique:	Exchanging Self-Portraits.	#14
Materials:	Paper and cray pas.	
Directions:	Draw a self-portrait and exchange for further additions; draw your partner and exchange.	
Population:	Married couples.	
Issues:	How I see you and perceive you; where we differ in opinion.	
Therapist:	Harriet Wadeson.	

Technique:	Physical Release of Anger.	#15
Materials:	Beanbag chair and tennis raquet.	
Directions:	Breathe deeply, allow sound to come out, and beat beanbag chair with tennis raquet.	
Population:	Child; adolescent; adult.	
Issues:	Release of anger, rage, physically to complement emotional art experience.	
Therapist:	Elaine Rapp.	

There is a natural flow from the feeling to the sensation world; before some patients can feel they must learn how to touch and become re-acquainted with their sensorium. The art therapist should be particularly at home in this world, as it is an intrinsic part of her sense of creative identification.

Sensation

Stimulation to my eyes and hands and imagination. Colors flowing—red, orange, magenta; now the silk touch of plaster warm and liquid against the rocky roughness of a hard and cold cast. Cold reception from a roomful of classmates or cold aching in my gut? NOW. Textures of stone, metal, yarn and steel wool. How do they make me feel? What images meet and flow with sensations to tell me more about me and being alive?

FUNCTION:	*Revealing*	FOCUS:	*Sensation*
Technique:	Meditative Drawing.		#1
Materials:	Paper and markers.		
Directions:	Close your eyes, relax and concentrate on bodily sensations. Stay with body awareness until you have clear images; draw abstractly to communicate your experience.		
Population:	Adolescent; adult.		
Issues:	Ability to quiet outer world and listen to inner world; sensitivity to sensorium.		
Therapist:	Efrem Weitzman.		
Technique:	Swallow a pea....		#2
Materials:	None.		
Directions:	Pretend to swallow a pea (or a Polaroid or a submarine) and verbally report where it is going and what it experiences within your body. Please exercise with caution.		
Population:	Child; adolescent; adult.		
Issues:	Body sensation, anatomy, imagination.		
Therapist:	Helen Landgarten, Paulette Floyd.		
Technique:	Photo Landscapes.		#3
Materials:	A collection of photos of various landscapes, i.e., desert, snowy mountains, tropical island, village, arctic, city.		

Directions:	Choose a locale and spin a fantasy of what appeals to you: what you do there, how life would be, etc.
Population:	Open.
Issues:	Environmental effects on emotions, temperatures, activities patient feels comfortable with.
Therapist:	Ginna Cottrell.

Technique:	Drawing to Music.	#4
Materials:	Records or tapes, paper and markers.	
Directions:	Listen for images, movement, colors, and draw what you see with eyes closed; abstract, loose, playful, serious. Bach, Beatles. Tibetan Bells.	
Population:	Open.	
Issues:	Coordination of rhythms, movement and auditory stimulus.	
Therapist:	Deborah Knable.	

Technique:	Moving Through Peanut Butter.	#5
Materials:	Paper and markers.	
Directions:	Imagine you are moving through peanut butter, jello, bubble gum, a roomful of pins, marbles, jungle, feathers, etc. Act out and draw sensations.	
Population:	Child.	
Therapist:	Cynthia Smith.	

Technique:	Ceramics.	#6
Materials:	Clay, clay tools, perhaps a wheel.	
Directions:	Handbuilding and throwing simple pots.	
Population:	Child; adolescent; adult.	
Issues:	Sensitivity to earthen clay and its various forms and states. Patience, being centered; an original product.	
Therapist:	Deborah Green.	

Technique:	Play Dough	#7
Materials:	Flour, salt, food coloring, water, plastic bag.	
Directions:	1 part salt mixed with 2 parts flour and colored water will give usable play clay. Good for play food. Can be baked in the oven to dry.	
Population:	Child, school or hospital.	
Issues:	Fun to mix from scratch, different feel of ingredients. Soft, coarse, wet, gushy, dry granular; measuring; stimulates fantasy.	
Therapist:	Joan Ellis.	

FUNCTION: *Revealing*   *FOCUS:*   *Sensation*

Technique: Sand Casting with Plaster.   #8
Materials: Sand in cardboard box, plaster of Paris, shells, junk.
Directions: Design in sand and pour in plaster.
Population: Child.
Issues: Contrasting textures, immediacy of product, i.e., wall
                hanging, mirror frame, abstract sculpture; messy but
                washes off.
Therapist: Deborah Green.

Technique: Finger Exercises.   #9
Materials: A partner.
Directions: Sitting cross-legged facing each other, eyes closed, join
                hands and stroke, poke, push, pull, caress, lift, clap.
Population: Adolescent; adult.
Issues: How much can you learn about another person only
                through the way he touches?
Therapist: Ilana Rubenfeld.

Technique: Touch Boxes.   #10
Materials: Shoe box, feathers, SOS, wire, fur, jello, gum, foil, etc.
Directions: Create a mini-environment within a shoe box that de-
                scribes your personality. Share it with others, their eyes
                closed. Get the message?
Population: Adult.
Issues: Sense perception connected to emotional awareness.
Therapist: Pratt Group Art Therapy class.

Technique: Cracker Collage.   #11
Materials: Half dozen different kinds of crackers, i.e. graham, Triskit,
                pretzel, Ritz, rye; cardboard and glue.
Directions: Make a collage, either representational or abstract.
Population: Child.
Issues: Textures and, undoubtedly, tastes.
Therapist: Linda Beth Sibley.

As was pointed out earlier, some patients need to order and logically think through their self-discovery process. Feeling and sensing are not enough; they must know and understand. A cognitive orientation to the often seemingly irregular evolution of growth can be facilitated through some of the following techniques.

Thinking

Logic dictates: I began with A and followed it with B and C;
WHY? why? why? Explaining me to myself; I began here and was
influenced by and got caught and then moved on. Why? This is my
story. I can record my growth and therefore understand it more fully.
Neat. Orderly. Rational. Explicable. Please clarify and describe that
better, for I need all the facts.

FUNCTION:	*Revealing*	FOCUS:	*Thinking*

Technique: Self Winnicott Scribble.   #1
Materials: Paper and markers.
Directions: Close your eyes, scribble for one minute, open and find
an image and develop it within the scribble.
Population: Adolescent; adult.
Issues: What image means to you, relevance to your life; what
does it tell you about conscious conflicts?
Therapist: Lynne Flexner Berger.

Technique: Cartoon Mural.   #2
Materials: Mural paper, markers and cray pas
Directions: Divide mural into 8 boxes of 8 patients and ask them to
draw within their own space a response to a given theme.
Population: Adult, psychotic.
Issues: Need for structure and safety within limited area.
Therapist: Linda Brown.

Technique: Mythology.   #3
Materials: Drawing materials and clay.
Directions: Define identifications with personal heroes and villains:
Snoopy, Batman, The Hulk. Draw, sculpt and act out a
scenario.
Population: Children.
Issues: Fantasy becoming real and experiential.
Therapist: Joan Columbus.

Technique: Journal of thoughts, dreams or perceptions.   #4
Materials: Blank book, drawing utensils and collage materials.
Directions: Keep a record of your personal growth via daily, weekly
entries, written and visual stories.
Population: Adult.
Issues: Respect for inner world; define patterns, continuity.
Therapist: Janie Rhyne (8).

FUNCTION:	*Revealing*	FOCUS:	*Thinking*
Technique:	My Necessities and Luxuries.		#5
Materials:	Mural paper and markers.		
Directions:	Draw all the things you need—then all the things you want.		
Population:	Adult, neurotic.		
Issues:	Separation of fantasy and reality; are necessities people, space, things, travel, food, attention?		
Therapist:	Elaine Rapp.		

Technique:	Lifeline.	#6
Materials:	Shelf paper, or adding machine rolls and markers.	
Directions:	Draw your life in images from birth until now and, perhaps, beyond. Time limit, i.e., half hour or an hour.	
Population:	Adolescent; adult, neurotic.	
Issues:	Space attributed to what events or emotions? What was omitted? Cause and effect clearer? Patterns evident?	
Therapist:	Janie Rhyne (8).	

Technique:	Faces.	#7
Materials:	Construction paper circles, crayons.	
Directions:	Make a face on the circle of paper.	
Population:	Adult, psychotic.	
Issues:	Acknowledgment of identity, expression.	
Therapist:	Linda Brown.	

Some patients need to be able to listen to themselves and trust their unconscious. They must first get in touch with a whole reservoir of images, fantasies and myths that lie somewhere in the pre-conscious recesses of the psyche. To learn how to listen to inner thoughts and phantoms and not be threatened by the strangeness of primary process thinking is extremely important. At times this falls into the nebulous category of intuition. There are a number of developmental tasks and exercises that highlight this area.

Intuition

I can read A and B and already know Y and Z, being able to use imagination and follow it wherever it may go. Trusting my hunches, clues that seem irrational (no one would believe I *knew* it before it happened!). Possibilities and probabilities. Hard to decide even the smallest thing. Ways of relying on answers that come up from inside without explanations and logic. What if . . . . ? ? ? Fantasies, you call them, but my realities. Implicit. Maybe mystical. Invisible but real.

FUNCTION:	*Revealing*	FOCUS:	*Intuition*

Technique:	Guided Image Trips.	#1
Materials:	Uninterrupted space, quiet, paper and markers.	
Directions:	T tells a story consisting mainly of images; P listens, responds and finally draws what he saw in his mind's eye. Example: meditation and visualization aiding in achieving a remission in cancer patients.	
Population:	Child; adolescent; adult, hospital.	
Issues:	Healing power of images.	
Therapist:	Dr. Carl Simonton, Michael Bova.	

Technique:	Magic Shop.	#2
Materials:	Space, quiet, paper and markers.	
Directions:	"You are lying on a beach in the hot sun, you go for a walk and find an old village. A small charming shop catches your eye. It's a magic shop and wonderful things are inside. Let your imagination wander and see what you find."	
Population:	Adult, neurotic.	
Issues:	What did you find? Temperature? Anything recognizable?	
Therapist:	Ilana Rubenfeld.	

Technique:	Magic Body/Magic Eyes.	#3
Materials:	Space, quiet, paper and markers.	
Directions:	Be the $6,000,000 man (kid) and make your body do anything you want. Where? What? How? What do you see?	
Population:	Child, hyperactive.	
Issues:	Identifying fantasies and wishes.	
Therapist:	David Davis, Susan Mann.	

Technique:	Original Plays and Masks.	#4
Materials:	Paper bags and paint.	
Directions:	Responses to a House-Tree-Person test became a play; characters come alive with the use of paper bag masks.	
Population:	Child.	

FUNCTION: *Revealing*   FOCUS: *Intuition*
Issues: Need to assimilate material brought up in testing
                    through imaginative acting-out.
Therapist: Linda Beth Sibley.

Technique: Change Your Dream.   #5
Materials: Recent dream, paper, markers and clay.
Directions: Verbally and visually create a more satisfactory ending
                    to an unhappy dream.
Population: Adolescent; adult.
Issues: Freedom and responsibility to create own reality.
Therapist: Elaine Kirson.

Technique: Storytelling.   #6
Materials: Popular story, myth, fable, i.e., "The Ant and the Grass-
                    hopper."
Directions: Read the story and ask P to change the ending; read
                    until the climax and ask for an original ending.
Population: Child.
Issues: Trusting one's own originality, power, foresight.
Therapist: Richard Gardner, Katherine Cripps (9).

Technique: Free Association Drawings.   #7
Materials: Paper and markers, pastels.
Directions: Draw anything and verbalize any thoughts and feelings.
Population: Child; adolescent; adult.
Issues: Comfort anxiety or inability to draw and verbalize im-
                    pulses, fantasies, associations; willingness to open up;
                    demonstrate trust.
Therapist: Myra Levick (7a).

All four of the above foci are aimed at learning to experience and know oneself better, trusting one's strengths and becoming wary of weaker and underdeveloped functions.

INTEGRATION

Integration of the self describes the third major category. These techniques are characterized neither by their emphasis on survival tools nor on analytic insights; they highlight all four areas of perception and judgment. Perhaps we could say these techniques are aimed at realizations about to become conscious within the patient. In each of the following techniques the processes within and without are strikingly parallel. The bridge connecting within and without is very short; the tension of energy crossing and recrossing this bridge is alive and vital. This is true for all kinds of patients—autistic children, acting-out adolescents and mature analysands. Immediacy, relevance and painfully obvious parallels seem to be the most distinguishing qualities of the following techniques. The focus here differentiates between techniques applied more successfully to either an individual patient or a group of patients.

FUNCTION:	*Integration*	*FOCUS:*	*Individual*
Technique:	Body Outline.		#1
Materials:	Mural paper or sheet and markers.		
Directions:	1. Lie down on paper on floor and trace body for another.		
	2. Name body parts as traced, label after for children.		
	3. Color in or fill with collage materials.		
Population:	Open.		
Issues:	Inner and outer image of physical self.		
Therapist:	Joan Ellis.		

Technique:	Draw Your Breath.	#2
Materials:	Paper and pencils.	
Directions:	T marks a dot on paper and asks P to start by drawing his breath.	
Population:	Adult, psychotic.	
Issues:	Encouragement for small energy expense, on paper and in relationship with T; a beginning.	
Therapist:	Joel Barg.	

Technique:	Pinch Pot.	#3
Materials:	Clay.	
Directions:	Form clay ball the size of your fist, push thumb down the center, pinch thumb against fingers while rotating ball. Try and stay centered so pot becomes balanced.	
Population:	Child; adolescent; adult.	
Issues:	Centering inside and out.	
Therapist:	Paulus Berensohn (10).	

FUNCTION:	*Integration*	*FOCUS:*	*Individual*

Technique: Poetry's Images.   #4
Materials: Original poetry, or Whitman, Sandburg, Gibran; paper and inks.
Directions: Read poetry aloud and illustrate.
Population: Adult, geriatric.
Issues: Feelings translated into words and images.
Therapist: Gloria Martin.

Technique: Ragdolls.   #5
Materials: Old sheets, scissors, yarn, doll pattern, scrap fabric, cotton stuffing.
Directions: Trace pattern, cut out, sew edges, turn and stuff. Add yarn hair and doll clothes.
Population: Adolescent, pregnant.
Issues: Manifestation of invisible body process.
Therapist: Nan Tesser, Ginna Cottrell.

Technique: Mandala.   #6
Materials: Paper, cray pas, paper plate and kaleidoscope.
Directions: Trace circle from plate, start in center and draw a balanced, centered design. Close eyes and watch colors and images. Use kaleidoscope for Ps stuck for impetus.
Population: Adult, psychiatric hospital.
Issues: Centering, balancing, meaning of images.
Therapist: Joan Kellogg.

Technique: Comic Book Cartoons, TV Pad.   #7
Materials: Hardcover drawing book, pencils.
Directions: P draws characters, T draws dialogue to create continuing story.
Population: Child, mute.
Issues: Messages from within become without.
Therapist: Michael Filan.

Technique: Clay Marionettes.   #8
Materials: Clay and wire.
Directions: Movable clay marionette made to resemble P; environment to scale.
Population: Adolescent, amputee.
Issues: Accepting physical reality through transitional object.
Therapist: Paulette Floyd.

Technique:	Ceramic Portraits.	#9
Materials:	Clay and a shoebox.	
Directions:	Make a relief portrait inside the shoebox, allow to dry, paint.	
Population:	Child, schizophrenic.	
Issues:	Ability to see self reflected within a limited, focused, safe, confined space.	
Therapist:	Deborah Green.	

Technique:	Doll House Series.	#10
Materials:	Cardboard, stones, plaster, paint.	
Directions:	Make three-dimensional houses representing various stages of identification, i.e., grandparents, parents, foster parents, child's residence.	
Population:	Child, orphan.	
Issues:	Foster parents, child's residence. House as interior structure of psyche.	
Therapist:	Dinah Kalin.	

Technique:	Polaroid Photographs.	#11
Materials:	Colorpak II camera.	
Directions:	Take picture of child and let him take pictures of his environment.	
Population:	Child, autistic.	
Issues:	Focusing and stabilizing self in immediate reality, physical and psychic.	
Therapist:	Ellen Nelson-Gee.	

Technique:	Zen and Painting.	#12
Materials:	Paper and paints.	
Directions:	Select an object (i.e., flower, chair) and imagine yourself becoming the essence of that object. Draw during or after.	
Population:	Adolescent; adult.	
Issues:	Centering, focusing within and without.	
Therapist:	Gloria Martin.	

Technique:	Stonecarving.	#13
Materials:	Stone, eyeshield, water bucket, pick and hammer.	
Directions:	Follow the flow of the stone and evolve sculpture.	
Population:	Adolescent; adult.	
Issues:	Internal dialogue, resistance, flexibility.	
Therapist:	Elaine Rapp.	

FUNCTION: *Integration*   FOCUS: *Individual*
Technique: Cakebox.   #14
Materials: Bakery cakebox, scissors, and markers.
Directions: Illustrate child self/adult self on the inside and outside
                  of the box; inner world and outer world; how you are and
                  how you would like to be, etc. Fashion into a paper
                  sculpture.
Population: Adult, neurotic.
Issues: Polarities and integration.
Therapist: Elaine Rapp.

Technique: Survey of Past Work.   #15
Materials: All art work drawn at a specific period of therapy.
Directions: At appropriate time, review art work.
Population: Adult, psychiatric hospital; private practice.
Issues: Cognition and integration of process.
Therapist: Myra Levick (7a).

Technique: Stencils.   #16
Materials: Tempera, paper, and scissors.
Directions: Cut stencil for P to paint in eye or nose, etc. rather than
                  paint for him.
Population: Child, mentally retarded.
Issues: Reaffirm worth of P, independence.
Therapist: Rosalind Seldigs.

Groups

Art therapists more often than not work with groups and require
a tremendous amount of grounding in group dynamics. There are
various group projects that highlight the interpersonal world of the
patient in a group and help facilitate dynamic interaction.

FUNCTION: *Integration*   FOCUS: *Groups*
Technique: Ethnic Music and Mural.   #1
Materials: Ethnic music, paper and pastels.
Directions: Listen, dance, share experiences of homeland and draw.
Population: Adult, psychiatric hospital.
Issues: Owning, appreciating and sharing one's heritage.
Therapist: Estelle Bellomo.

Technique:	Blind/Sound Floor Mural.	#2
Materials:	Mural paper and pastels.	
Directions:	Place mural and pastels on floor; eyes closed, make a sound and draw to that sound for ten minutes. Open eyes and elaborate design.	
Population:	Adult, neurotic.	
Issues:	Primitive sound relatedness, vibrations, movement, space.	
Therapist:	Michael Edwards.	

Technique:	My Name.	#3
Materials:	Paper and markers.	
Directions:	Dramatically enunciate your name; match syncopated sound with appropriate body movement. No name tags; identify other group members by their sound and body language.	
Population:	Adult, neurotic. Clear statement of individual identity opens door for group identity formation.	
Therapist:	Christopher Beck.	

Technique:	Clay Figures.	#4
Materials:	Clay.	
Directions:	Model a figure of another group member in a posture that clearly communicates his feeling.	
Population:	Adult, prison inmates.	
Issues:	Body language as a reflection of one's inner world.	
Therapist:	Jan Adler, Dina Rose.	

Technique:	Treasured Objects.	#5
Materials:	Personal belonging.	
Directions:	Ask each P to bring his most precious possession. Share its meaning and related experience.	
Population:	Adult, geriatric.	
Issues:	Self disclosure, past becoming present.	
Therapist:	Gloria Martin.	

COMBINATION TECHNIQUES

Several techniques can be used for *Building Out, Revealing* and/or *Integrating,* depending on utilization by the therapist and her view

of a particular patient. A few such versatile, "open-ended" techniques
are listed here.

FUNCTION:	*All*	FOCUS:	*Open*

Technique:	Super 8 Films, Filmstrips, Slide Series	#1
Materials:	Appropriate equipment.	
Directions:	Write, animate, edit and show film as illustration of folk song, fable or myth.	
Population:	Adolescent, psychiatric hospital.	
Issues:	Planning, frustration tolerance, coordination of music and imagery, cooperation.	
Therapist:	Jeff Goshen.	

Technique:	Videotape and Polaroid Camera.	#2
Materials:	Appropriate equipment.	
Directions:	1. Tape a therapy encounter, use with psychodrama or write a story and act out for TV.	
	2. Photograph group interactions.	
Population:	Child; adolescent; adult	
Issues:	Immediacy of self-image via objective ego of camera.	
Therapist:	Milton M. Berger (11), Ellen Nelson-Gee.	

Technique:	Poetry.	#3
Materials:	Books of favorite poetry, paper and pencils. Read a classic and illustrate, i.e., Blake, Cummings.	
Directions:	Read a poem and write a poetic response. Choose a fantasy topic and write your own poem.	
Population:	Child; adolescent; adult.	
Issues:	Imagery's relation to feelings through works and/or pictures.	
Therapist:	Morris Morrison, Pierre Boenig.	

Technique:	Collection of Objects.	#4
Materials:	Miniature houses, matchbox cars, keys, hats—any group of similar but individually distinctive objects.	
Directions:	Choose a key and fantasize the door it opens; choose a house and fantasize who lives in it.	
Population:	Adolescent; adult.	
Issues:	Resonate with an image and own it; explore your fantasies.	
Therapist:	Elaine Rapp.	

Technique:	Sequential Graphics.	#5
Materials:	Shelf paper or notebook or small pads and markers.	

Directions:	Series of drawings that tells a story.
	1. P draws all.
	2. P and T take turns drawing.
	3. T draws problem and P draws solution.
	4. Group shares in creating a story.
Population:	Child; adolescent; adult, mute.
Issues:	Quick movement of story, minimum drawing skill required.
Therapist:	Bernard Stone.

Technique:	Sandplay.	#6
Materials:	Sandbox 19″ × 29″ and miniature figures of animals, people. Without sand, clay flattened into a pancake acts as a base.	
Directions:	Make a picture and tell a story.	
Population:	Child; adult.	
Issues:	Safety within limits of the box, picture reflects intrapsychic forces.	
Therapist:	Dora Kalff.	

Technique:	Family Art Therapy.	#7
Materials:	Easels, large pads, and pastels for each member.	
Directions:	Draw and title:	
	1. Free drawing.	
	2. Family portrait.	
	3. Abstract family portrait.	
	4. Eyes closed drawing.	
	5. Scribble.	
	6. Joint family scribble.	
	7. Free drawing.	
Issues:	Families—therapist should observe art product, behavior and verbal interaction.	
Therapist:	Hanna Kwiatkowska.	

Technique:	Psychodrama.	#8
Materials:	None.	
Directions:	Role-play yourself and/or others in emotional situations.	
Population:	Adolescent; adult.	
Issues:	Open expression of feelings, problem solving.	
Therapist:	Hanna Weiner.	

Technique:	Multimedia.	#9
Materials:	Non-destructible room, piano, tape recorder, telephone, music, junk, art materials, and total freedom.	

FUNCTION: *All*   FOCUS: *Open*
Directions: Explore possibilities offered here; no limits.
Population: Adolescent, residence.
Issues: Choice, freedom and responsibility.
Therapist: Susan Swamm.

Technique: Communicators.   #10
Materials: Telephone, tape recorder, walkie talkie (real, toy or
                 home made).
Directions: Imagine conversations or letters—telling people off or
                 turning people on.
Population: Adolescent.
Issues: Practice in communicating, appeal of machines, audio
                 reflection.
Therapist: Bob Wolf.

We conclude our survey with four of the most commonly used projective techniques which comprise an art experience designed to divulge information not directly obtainable from the patient or case records.

Handled with care, the therapist can emphasize the "fantasy-play" aspect over that of the "testing" element that so often seems antitherapeutic (12).

FUNCTION: *Gathering Information*   FOCUS: *Open*
Technique: Scribble Drawings.   #1
Materials: Paper and crayons.
Directions: T scribbles and P makes an image; P scribbles and T
                 makes an image.
Population: Child.
Issues: Rapport builder, fun, significant images surface, drawing
                 becomes transitional object.
Therapist: D. W. Winnicott (13).

Technique: Draw-A-Person Test.   #2
Materials: Typing paper and No. 2 pencil.
Directions: 1. Draw a person.
                 2. Draw a person of the opposite sex. T follows through
                    with post-drawing questionnaire and evaluation.
Population: Child; adult.
Issues: Self-image, sexual identification.
Therapist: Karen Machover (14).

Technique:	House-Tree-Person Test.	#3
Materials:	Typing paper and No. 2 pencil.	
Directions:	1. Draw a house.	
	2. Draw a tree.	
	3. Draw a person.	
	T follows through with post-drawing questionnaire and evaluation.	
Population:	Child; adult.	
Issues:	Self-image, fantasy life.	
Therapist:	John S. Buck (15).	

Technique:	Kinetic Family Drawing Test.	#4
Materials:	Typing paper and No. 2 pencil.	
Directions:	Draw a family doing something.	
Population:	Child; adult.	
Issues:	Interpersonal dynamics of P's family.	
Therapist:	Robert Burns and S. H. Kaufman (16).	

No chapter on techniques would be complete if we did not mention that art is often used in conjunction with other modalities, i.e., music, dance, movement and even sports. To move with music while expressing oneself graphically allows the art therapist to broaden the range of the way she touches sense and relates to people. There will be many art therapists who will be reluctant to broaden their horizons to integrate dance and music into their repertoire. But as pressure increases to unify the various expressive modalities and break through artificial restrictions, the therapist will be increasingly strong in her position if she does not restrict herself solely to graphic techniques. Music in the background, movement of colors, the rhythm of forms all imply that a patient cannot be compartmentalized or relegated to a dance, drama, art or music therapist.

In sum, our underlying thesis is one of openness to the challenge of each situation and the inherent demands of the patient population, institution and specific talents of the individual therapist. Creativity is our stock in trade. Can we afford to be inflexible?

References

1. Kandinsky, D. "The Meaning of Technique." *Journal of Analytical Psychology*. Vol. 15, 165–176, 1970.

2. Plaut, A. "What Do You Actually Do? Problems in Communicating about Analytic Technique." *Journal of Analytical Psychology*. Vol. 15, 13–22, 1970.

3. Wolberg, L. *The Technique of Psychotherapy*. 2 vols. New York: Grune & Stratton, 1967.

4. Menninger, K. *Theory of Psychoanalytic Technique*. New York: Basic Books, 1958.

5. *Bulletin of Art Therapy*. Fall 1961–July 1969.

6. *American Journal of Art Therapy*, Vol. 1–13: October 1969–January 1974.

7. Denny, J. M. "Techniques for Individual and Group Art Therapy." *American Journal of Art Therapy*. Vol. 11 (3): April 1972.

7a. Fink, P., Levick, M., and Vaccaro, M. (Eds.) *Dynamic Art Therapy and Its Applications*. New York: Teachers College Press, in preparation.

8. Rhyne, J. *The Gestalt Art Experience*. Monterey, California: Brooks/Cole, 1973.

9. Gardner, R. *Therapeutic Consultations With Children: The Mutual Story Telling Technique*. New York: Spence House, 1971.

10. Berensohn, P. *Finding One's Way with Clay*. New York: Simon and Schuster, 1968.

11. Berger, M. M. *Videotape Techniques in Psychiatric Training and Treatment*. New York: Brunner/Mazel, 1970.

12. Hammer, E. F. *The Clinical Application of Projective Drawings*. Springfield, Ill. Charles C Thomas, 1967.

13. Winnicott, D. W. *Therapeutic Consultations in Child Psychiatry*. New York: Basic Books, 1971.

14. Machover, K. A. *Personality Projection in the Drawing of the Human Figure: A Method of Personality Investigation*. Springfield, Ill. Charles C Thomas, 1957.

15. Buck, J. S. *The House-Tree-Person Techniques*. Los Angeles: Western Psychological Services, 1966.

16. Burns, R. C., and Kaufman, S. H. *Kinetic Family Drawings. (K-F-D): An Introduction to Understanding Children Through Kinetic Drawings*. New York: Brunner/Mazel, 1970.

APPENDIX A
INTERVIEW FORM

1. Name.
2. Address.
3. Telephone.
4. School or training program for art therapy.
5. Other related training.
6. Any therapy of your own (optional).
7. Years practicing art therapy.
8. Field work placement or employing institution.
9. Theoretical approach and/or book that most influenced you.
10. Physical and/or psychic state of patient.
11. Age.
12. Individual or group.
13. How often seen.
14. Quality of interpersonal connection.
15. Describe therapeutic impasse/problem and how you creatively solved it with an art therapy technique.
16. Applicable to other patient populations.
17. Comments.

APPENDIX B
QUESTIONNAIRE

My name is Linda Sibley. My master's thesis is to be a collection of art therapy techniques currently being used by students and professionals in our field. The result will hopefully be a book that will act as a reference for all of us. Would you be kind enough to fill out this questionnaire? I would like to interview everyone personally but because of time will not be able to. If you would prefer to talk to me by phone, please indicate below. This questionnaire may be returned to me or left in the art therapy office. Many thanks for your cooperation.

Name_____

Telephone_____ Phone interview?_____

Field work placement_____

Training besides Pratt_____

Years practicing art therapy_____

Had any therapy of your own?_____ What kind_____

Define your own theoretical approach_____

★★★

Setting you work in _____

Individual or group_____

Sex or client_____ Age _____

Physical state _____

How often do you see client? _____

Any auxiliary factors? (environment, recent crisis) _____

Define the quality of your connection to the client. (Tension, affectionate, friendly, angry) _____ _____

Do you work alone or with co-therapists?_____

Anything else relevant that I should know to define the situation where the specific technique you describe might be used?

_____

_____

When you are faced with a problem, a resistance, an impasse or when you are stuck, when the flow of creative energy between yourself and your client comes to a halt, what do you do? How do you use humor? How do you redirect hostility? How do you build a better body image? Release tension? Allow anger? Explain racial prejudice? Explain sex? Offer emotional sup-

250

port? Increase sensory awareness? With smells, textures, tastes? Do you use sports or cooking and for what therapeutic goal? How do you move from fantasy to reality? What materials used beyond paint and clay?

These are the kind of questions that might be helpful in clarifying what I mean by technique. I am looking for exactly what you do when you do art therapy and why you chose to make a specific approach. Try and think of a specific situation and describe it below.

★★★★★★★★★★★★★★★★★★★★★★★

Problem _____

_____

Your feeling and how experienced _____

_____

Client's feeling and how experienced _____

_____

Focus or goal for movement _____

_____

Describe the technique. What limits did you set? Time elapsed? Specific materials? What direction did you give? Verbal or nonverbal exercise?

_____

_____

_____

_____

_____

_____

_____

_____

_____

_____

_____

What was your response to the experience? _____
Client's response? _____
How did this exercise fit into the process of your relationship or the growth process of the client? _____

Has technique been tried with a different patient population and how effective was it? _____

_____

APPENDIX C
CONTRIBUTORS

Leslie Abrams
Robin Abramson
Janet Adler
Jan Adler
Robert Ault
Linda Axelrod
Nancy Bagel
Joel Barg
Christopher Beck
Estelle Bellomo
Paulus Berensohn
Lynne Flexner Berger
Milton M. Berger
Mala Betensky
Jessie Bighach
Pierre Boenig
Michael Bova
Linda Brown
John S. Buck
Robert Burns
George Carter
Harriet Cheney
Joan Columbus
Ginna Cottrell
Katherine Cripps
Shellie David
David Davis
James Denny
Pamela Diamond
Roberta Dubinksy
Michael Edwards
Joan Ellis
Randy Faerber
Susan B. Fine
Michael Filan
Paulette Floyd
Olive Galdston
Theodora Garris

Richard Gardner
Pam Glick
Emory Gondor
Jeff Goshen
Rosemary Grassi
Deborah Green
Peggy Griffin
Toby Gross
Vicky Harris
Martha Hessler
Rachel Hickman
Julia Housekeeper
Cliff Joseph
Georgianna Jungels
Dinah Kahn
Dora Kalff
Barbara Katz
Marla Katz
S. H. Kaufman
Joan Kellogg
Hanna Kwiatkowska
Elaine Kirson
Deborah Knable
Helen Landgarten
Myra Levick
Janet Lewis
Eileen Lordahl
Jil Lustgarten
Karen Machover
Barbara Maciag
Susan Mann
Gloria Martin
Jane Morrin
Morris Morrison
Sonia Moscowitz
Constance Naitove
Ellen Nelson-Gee
Pat Newell-Hall

Deborah Oberfest
Penny Perelman
Madeleine Petrillo
Ben Ploger
Frances Plonsky
Elaine Rapp
Linc Reinhart
Janie Rhyne
Dina Rose
Mickie Rosen
Ilana Rubenfeld
Rosalind Seldigs
Seth H. Shaw
Linda Beth Sibley
Ellen Simon
Carl Simonton
Cynthia Smith
Mary Steele
Bernard Stone
Lee Straus
Susan Swamm
David Tavin
Nan Tesser
Leslie Thompson
Madeline Tisch
Eleanor Ulman
Harriet Wadeson
Ann Watson
Hanna Weiner
Bernard Weitzman
Efrem Weitzman
D. W. Winnicott
Maxine Whiteman
Bob Wolf
Cynthia Wolf
Wendy Wulbrandt

Conclusion

In many respects, art therapy can supply a missing dimension in education and psychotherapy. Both fields of late have become increasingly pragmatic and behavior oriented in their approach. These trends are an understandable reaction to a naïve, often simplistic, application of psychodynamic theory. However, in this reaction there lies a potential danger in overlooking the positive values of an orientation concerned with development of the inner being. Symptomatic release, mastery of skills and effective performance are goals that need not preclude, but may accompany, an inner search for one's self. All too often, the worlds of performance and self-development have become compartmentalized. Clinical evidence has long indicated a firm relationship between sensory, perceptual and cognitive growth (1). Enlightened art therapy practice can address itself to these multiple areas and offer an experience that helps the patient to deal effectively with the inner as well as the outer world.

The art therapist should not limit his creativity to a specific sphere but relate to a whole Gestalt of factors, utilizing his creativity wherever it is needed. The emerging art therapist needs to be in deep harmony not only with his patients, his community, and his art work, but also with himself. The pressures of society make adaptation and effective performance very respectable values while freedom to explore and play is seen as an attribute that belongs in the nursery. We trust art therapy will elevate the magic and wonder of the child's attitude to an equal place in productive and effective living. The inner self that can function on multiple levels of consciousness can lead to development of imaginative and creative skills. For some children and adults, the availability of a creative approach may mean actual survival.

Currently, art therapists are working in large metropolitan health care institutions. Some day, these new professionals may find more positions in the areas of industry and ecology. Bringing together knowledge of aesthetics, spatial relations and an openness to alternatives, and converting these to the needs of large organizations may be a future inroad for art therapy. As the creative counterparts to the modern-day social psychologist, art therapists may encourage the growth of an environment which is creatively playful, as well as one that maximizes effective adaptations.

In the future we see art therapy expanding as a profession in many different directions. Newer discoveries in the area of biofeedback may add another dimension to a psychological base that will give extra force and momentum to work with deeply disturbed patients (2). Recent studies into left and right cerebral specialization have exciting implications, and will stimulate research further in the field of creativity development (3). Collaboration with other expressive therapies, such as dance, movement, and music, has begun and shall continue for both increased political strength and more effective patient care (4). We see creative art therapy being structured and restructured constantly, as each new artist-therapist discovers herself professionally. Soon, we will return to this written text with fresh ideas that will inevitably arise as our dialogue in the creative process continues.

References

1. Arnheim, R. Visual Thinking. Berkeley: University of California Press, 1969.
2. Jonas, G. Biofeedback Training. New York: The Viking Press, 1973.
3. Ornstein, R. The Psychology of Human Consciousness. New York: The Viking Press, 1973.
4. In November of 1974, Mayor Beame of New York City declared "Creative Arts Therapies Week" as the Art, Dance, and Music Therapy Associations all held their annual national conventions there.

Bibliography

Adler, A. *The Practice and Theory of Individual Psychology*. Translated by P. Radin, New York: Harcourt, Brace, 1924.

Adler, G. *The Living Symbol: A Case Study in the Process of Individuation*. New York: Pantheon Books, 1961.

Alexander, F. and French, T. M. *Psychoanalytic Therapy*. New York: Ronald Press, 1944.

Anthony, J. A. and Koupernik, C. *The Child in His Family: The Impact of Disease and Death*. Vol. 2. New York: Wiley, 1973.

Altman, C. *The Dream in Psychoanalysis*. New York: International Universities Press, 1969.

American Journal of Art Therapy. Vol. 1–13: Washington, D.C.: October 1969–January 1974.

Arguelles, J. and Arguelles, M. *Mandala*. Berkeley, California: Shambala, 1972.

Arnheim, R. *Art and Visual Perception: A Psychology of Creative Eye*. Berkeley: University of California Press, 1954.

Arnheim, R. *Visual Thinking*. Berkeley: University of California Press, 1969.

Axline, Virginia. *Play Therapy*. New York: Ballantine Books, Revised Edition, 1969.

Barron, F. X. *Creativity and Personal Freedom*. Princeton, N.J.: Van Nostrand Reinhold, 1962.

Becket, L. C. *Movement, Exploration, and Games for the Mentally Retarded*. Palo Alto, California: Peek Publications, 1970.

Becket, P. *Adolescents out of Step: Their Treatment in a Psychiatric Hospital* New York: Basic Books, 1953.

Benime, W. *The Clinical Use of Dreams*. New York: Basic Books, 1962.

Berebin, M. *Geriatric Psychiatry*. New York: International Universities Press, 1967.

Berensohn, P. *Finding One's Way with Clay*. New York: Simon and Schuster, 1968.

Berger, M. *Videotape Techniques in Psychiatric Training and Treatment*. New York: Brunner/Mazel, 1970.

Berkowitz, I. H., Ed. *Adolescents Grow in Groups*. New York: Brunner/Mazel, 1972.

Birch, H. *Brain Damage in Children*. Baltimore: Williams & Wilkins, 1964.

Birren, F. *Color Psychology and Color Therapy: A Factual Study of the Influence of Color on Human Life*. New York: McGraw-Hill, 1950.

Bloss, P. *On Adolescence*. New York: Free Press, 1952.

Buck, J. S. *The House-Tree-Person Technique*. Los Angeles, California: Western Psychological Services, 1966.

Bulletin of Art Therapy. Washington, D.C.: Fall 1961–July 1969.

Burns, R. C. and Kaufman, S. H. *Kinetic Family Drawings.* (*K-F-D*): *An Introduction to Understanding Children Through Kinetic Drawings.* New York: Brunner/Mazel, 1970.

Burton, E. W. *Psychotherapy of the Psychosis.* New York: Basic Books, 1961.

Bychowski, G. "Struggle Against the Introjects." *International Journal of Psychoanalysis.* Vol. 39, 83–91, 1958.

Cane, F. *The Artist in Each of Us.* New York: Pantheon Books, 1951.

Caplan, F. and Caplan, T. *The Power of Play.* Garden City, New York: Anchor Press/Doubleday, 1974.

Castillejo, I. C. de. *Knowing Woman.* New York: Harper and Row, 1973.

Cirlot, J. E. *A Dictionary of Symbols.* Translated by Jack Sage. New York: Philosophical Library, 1972.

Colby, K. M. *A Primer for Psychotherapists.* New York: Ronald Press, 1951.

Denny, James M. "Techniques for Individual and Group Art Therapy." *American Journal of Art Therapy.* Vol. 11 (3), 91–98, April 1972.

Deutsch, F. and Murphy, W. *The Clinical Interview.* New York: International Universities Press, 1963.

DiLeo, J. H. *Young Children and Their Drawings.* New York: Brunner/Mazel, 1970.

Ehrenzweig, A. *The Hidden Order of Art: A Study in the Psychology of Artistic Imagination.* Berkeley: University of California Press, 1967.

Ekstein, R. *Children of Space and Time: Action and Impulses.* New York: International Universities Press, 1965.

Eliade, M. *Shamanism.* Princeton: Princeton University Press, 1964.

Ellenberger, H. F. *The Discovery of the Unconscious.* New York: Basic Books, 1970.

Engel, M. *Psychopathology in Children: Social, Diagnostic and Therapeutic Aspects.* New York: Harcourt, Brace, Jovanovich, 1972.

Erikson, E. *Childhood and Society.* New York: International Universities Press, 1956.

Evan, T. W., *Brain Injured Children.* Springfield, Illinois: Charles C Thomas, 1969.

Fairbairn, U. R. D. *An Object Relations Theory of the Personality.* New York: Basic Books, 1958.

Fenichel, O. *The Psychoanalytic Theory of Neurosis.* New York: W. W. Norton, 1945.

Fraiberg, S. *The Magic Years.* New York: Charles Scribner Sons, 1959.

Freud, A. *Normalcy and Pathology in Children.* New York: International Universities Press, 1965.

Freud, A. *The Ego and the Mechanisms of Defense.* New York: International Universities Press, 1967.

Freud, S. *A General Introduction to Psychoanalysis.* New York: Garden City Publishing, Doubleday, 1943.

Freud, S. *The Interpretation of Dreams.* Translated by Grill. New York: The Modern Library, 1950.

Freud, S. *On Creativity and the Unconscious; Papers on the Psychology of Art, Literature, Love, Religion.* New York: Harper, 1958.

Fromm-Reichman, F. *Principles of Intensive Psychotherapy.* Chicago, Illinois: University of Chicago Press, 1950.

Fromm, E. *The Forgotten Language.* New York: Grove Press, 1951.

Gantt, L. and Schmal, M. S. *Art Therapy: A Bibliography.* Washington, D.C.: National Institute of Mental Health, 1974.

Gardner, H. *The Arts and Human Development: A Psychological Study of the Artistic Process.* New York: Wiley, 1973.

Gardner, R. *Therapeutic Consultations with Children: The Mutual Story Telling Technique.* New York: Spence House, 1971.

Ginott, H. *Group Psychotherapy with Children.* New York: McGraw-Hill, 1961.

Glover, E. *The Technique of Psychoanalysis.* New York: International Universities Press, 1958.

Greenacre, P. *Affective Disorders.* New York: International Universities Press, 1953.

Greenacre, P. "Play in Relation to Creative Imagination." *Psychoanalytic Study of the Child.* Vol. XIV, 1959, New York: International Universities Press.

Greenberg, P. *Children's Experiences in Art: Drawings and Paintings.* New York: Van Nostrand Reinhold, 1966.

Greenwald, H. *Active Psychotherapy.* Chicago: Atherton Press, 1967.

Guggenbuhl-Craig, A. *Power in the Helping Professions.* New York: Spring Publications, 1971.

Haley, J. *Strategies of Psychotherapy.* New York: Grune & Stratton, 1963.

Hall, C. S., and Lindzey, G. *Theories of Personality.* New York: John Wiley and Sons, 1957.

Hammer, E. F. *The Clinical Application of Projective Drawings.* Springfield, Illinois: Charles C Thomas, 1967.

Harms, E. *Essentials of Abnormal Child Psychiatry.* New York: Julion Press, 1953.

Hartley, R. E. *The Complete Book of Children's Play.* Thomas C. Crowell, 1957.

Hatterer, L. J. *The Artist in Society: Problems and Treatment of the Creative Personality.* New York: Grove Press, 1965.

Horney, K. *The Collected Works of Karen Horney.* New York: W. W. Norton, 1964.

Jacobson, E. *The Self and the Object World.* New York: International Universities Press, 1964.

Jaeger, D., and Simos, L. *The Aged Ill.* New York: Meredith Eop., 1970.

Jonas, G. *Biofeedback Training.* New York: The Viking Press, 1973.

Jones, R. *The New Psychology of Dreams.* New York: Grune & Stratton, 1970.

Jung, C. G. *Mandala Symbolism.* Princeton: Bollingen Foundation, 1959.

Jung, C. G. *Memories, Dreams, Reflections.* Recorded and edited by Aniela Jaffe. New York: Pantheon Books, 1963.

Jung, C. G. *The Portable Jung.* Ed. J. Campbell. Translated R. F. C. Hull. New York: The Viking Press, 1971.

Kalff, D. M. *Sandplay*. San Francisco: Browser Press, 1971.

Kandinsky, D. "The Meaning of Technique." *Journal of Analytical Psychology*. Vol. 15, 165–176, 1970.

Kaplan, O. *Mental Disorder in Later Life*. Stanford, California: Stanford University Press, 1956.

Kellogg, R. *Analyzing Children's Art*. Palo Alto, California: National Press Books, 1969.

Kellogg, R., and O'Dell, S. *The Psychology of Children's Art*. New York: Random House, 1967.

Kelsey, M. T. *Dreams: The Dark Speech of the Spirit*. Garden City: Doubleday, 1968.

Koestler, A. *The Art of Creation*. New York: Macmillan, 1964.

Kramer, E. *Art as Therapy with Children*. New York: Schocken Books, 1972.

Kramer, E. *Art Therapy in a Children's Community*. Springfield, Illinois: Charles C Thomas, 1958.

Kris, E. *Psychoanalytic Explorations in Art*. New York: International Universities Press, 1952.

Kubie, L. S. *Neurotic Distortion of the Creative Process*. New York: Noonday Press, 1961.

Laing, R. D. *The Divided Self*. New York: Pantheon, 1969.

Laing, R. D. *The Politics of Experience*. New York: Pantheon, 1967.

Lazarus, A. *Clinical Behavior Therapy*. New York: Brunner/Mazel, 1972.

Levin, S., and Kabana, R. *Psychodynamic Studies on Aging—Creativity, Reminiscing and Dying*. New York: International Universities Press, 1967.

Linderman, E. W., and Herberholz, D. W. *Developing Artistic and Perceptual Awareness: Art Practice in the Elementary Classroom*. 2nd ed. Dubuque, Iowa: W. C. Brown, 1969.

Lindsay, Z. *Art and the Handicapped Child*. New York: Van Nostrand Reinhold, 1972.

Lindstrom, M. *Children's Art: A Study of Normal Development in Children's Modes of Visualization*. Berkeley: University of California Press, 1967.

Lowenfeld, V. *Creative and Mental Growth*. 6th ed. New York: Macmillan, 1975.

Lyddiatt, E. M. *Spontaneous Painting and Modelling: A Practical Approach in Therapy*. New York: St. Martin's Press, 1972.

Machover, K. A. *Personality Projection in the Drawing of the Human Figure: A Method of Personality Investigation*. 1st ed. Springfield, Illinois: Charles C Thomas, 1957.

Mahler, M. *On Human Symbiosis and the Vicissitudes of Individuation*. New York: International Universities Press, 1968.

Maslow, A. H. *The Creative Attitude*. New York: Psychosynthesis Research Foundation, 1963.

Maslow, A. H. *Toward a Psychology of Being*. New York: Van Nostrand Reinhold, 1968.

May, R. *Love and Will*. New York: W. W. Norton, 1969.

McDonald, J. L., and Bell, J. *Narcotic Addiction*. New York: Harper and Row, 1966.

Meares, A. *The Door of Serenity: A Study in the Therapeutic Use of Symbolic Painting.* London: Faber and Faber, 1958.

Menet, O., and French, J., Eds. *Psychiatric Approach to Mental Retardation.* New York: Basic Books, 1970.

Menninger, K. *Theory of Psychoanalytic Technique.* New York: Basic Books, 1958.

Milner, M. *On Not Being Able to Paint.* New York: International Universities Press, 1957.

Moustakas, C. E. *Psychotherapy with Children.* New York: Ballantine Books, 1959.

Naumburg, M. *Dynamically Oriented Art Therapy: Its Principles and Practices.* New York: Grune & Stratton, 1966.

Naumburg, M. *Psychoneurotic Art: Its Function in Psychotherapy.* New York: Grune & Stratton, 1953.

Naumburg, M. *Schizophrenic Art: Its Meaning in Psychotherapy.* New York: Grune & Stratton, 1950.

Naumburg, M. *Studies of the "Free" Art Expression of Behavior Problem Children and Adolescents as a Means of Diagnosis and Therapy.* New York: Coolidge Foundation, 1947.

Nelson, M. C., and Meerloe, J. *Transference and Trial Adoption.* Springfield, Illinois: Charles C Thomas, 1965.

Nelson, M., Nelson, B., Herman, M., and Stream, H. *Roles and Paradigms in Psychotherapy.* New York: Grune & Stratton, 1968.

Neumann, E. *Art and the Creative Unconscious: Four Essays.* New York: Princeton University Press, 1969.

Nicolaides, K. *The Natural Way to Draw.* Boston: Houghton, Mifflin, 1941.

Ornstein, R. *The Psychology of Human Consciousness.* New York: The Viking Press, 1973.

Perls, F. S. *Gestalt Therapy Verbatim.* Lafayette, California: Real People Press, 1969.

Petrillo, M., and Sanger, S. *Emotional Care of Hospitalized Children.* Philadelphia: Lippincott, 1972.

Pfister, O. R. *Expressionism in Art, Its Psychological and Biological Basis.* London: K. Paul, Trench, Trubner & Co., 1922.

Phillips, W., ed. *Art and Psychoanalysis.* Cleveland: World Pub. Co., 1963.

Pickford, R. W. *Studies in Psychiatric Art: Its Psychodynamics, Therapeutic Value and Relationship to Modern Art.* Springfield, Illinois: Charles C Thomas, 1967.

Plaut, A. "What Do You Actually Do? Problems in Communicating about Analytic Technique." *Journal of Analytical Psychology.* Vol. 15, 13–22, 1970.

Prinzhorn, H. *Artistry of the Mentally Ill: A Contribution to the Psychology and Psycho-Pathology of Configuration.* New York: Springer-Verlag, 1972.

Rank, O. *Art and Artist: Creative Urge and Personality Development.* New York: Agathon Press, 1968.

Rapp, E. *The Creative Growth Experience.* New York: 1971.

Reich, W. *Character Analysis.* New York: Simon and Schuster, 1945.

Reik, T. *Listening with the Third Ear*. New York: Pyramid Communications, 1948.

Rhyne, J. *The Gestalt Art Experience*. Monterey, California: Brooks/Cole, 1973.

Rie, H. E. *Perspectives in Child Psychopathology*. Chicago, Illinois: Alake-Atherton, 1971.

Rosen, J. *Direct Analysis*. New York: Grune & Stratton, 1953.

Ross, E. K. *On Death and Dying*. New York: Macmillan, 1969.

Sachs, H. *The Creative Unconscious: Studies in the Psychoanalysis of Art*. 2nd enl. ed., Cambridge, Massachusetts: Sci-Art Publishers, 1951.

Satir, V. *Conjoint and Family Therapy*. New York: Science and Behavior Books, Inc., 1967.

Saunders, R. J. *Art for the Mentally Retarded in Connecticut*. Hartford, Connecticut: Connecticut State Department of Education, 1967.

Schafer, Roy. *Aspects of Internalization*. New York: International Universities Press, 1968.

Scott, I. A. (Ed. and Translator). *The Luscher Color Test*. New York: Random House, 1969.

Searles, H. *The Non-Human Environment*. New York: International Universities Press, 1960.

Searles, H. *Colletced Papers on Schizophrenia*. New York: International Universities Press, 1965.

Sechehaye, M. A. *Symbolic Realization*. New York: International Universities Press, 1960.

Senn, M. J. E., and Solnit, A. J. *Problems in Child Behavior and Development*. Philadelphia: Lea and Febiger, 1968.

Sharpe, E. F. *Dream Analysis*. London: Hogarth Press, 1937.

Sullivan, H. S. *The Interpersonal Theory of Psychiatry*. 1st ed. New York: Norton & Co., 1953.

Sunderland, J. T. *Older Americans and the Arts*. Washington, D.C.: Public National Center for the Arts and Aging, undated.

Suzuki, D. T. Fromm, E., and De Martino, R. *Zen Buddhism and Psychoanalysis*. New York: Grove Press, 1962.

Szasz, T. *The Myth of Mental Illness*. New York: Harper, 1961.

Tarachow, S. *An Introduction to Psychotherapy*. New York: International Universities Press, 1963.

Teilhard de Chardin, P. *The Phenomenon of Man*. New York: Harper and Row, 1959.

Torrance, P. E. *Guiding Creative Talent*. Englewood Cliffs, N.J.: Prentice Hall, 1963.

Uhlin, D. M. *Art for Exceptional Children*. Dubuque, Iowa: W. C. Brown, 1972.

Waelder, R. *Psychoanalytic Avenues to Art*. New York: International Universities Press, 1965.

Wickes, F. G. *The Inner World of Childhood: A Study in Analytical Psychology*. New York: Appleton-Century, 1966.

Winnicott, D. W. *Therapeutic Consultations in Child Psychiatry.* New York: Basic Books, 1971.

Winnicott, D. W. *Through Paediatrics to Psycho-Analysis.* New York: Basic Books, 1975.

Wolberg, L. *The Technique of Psychotherapy.* New York: Grune & Stratton, 1967.

Wolpe, J., and Lazarus, A. A. *Behavior Therapy Techniques.* New York: Pergamon Press, 1966.